ABC of
Cancer Care

ABC series

An outstanding collection of resources for everyone in primary care

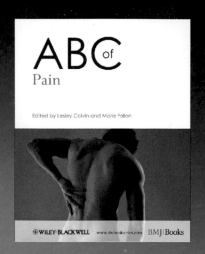

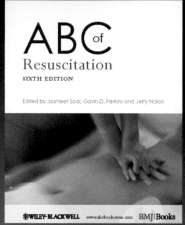

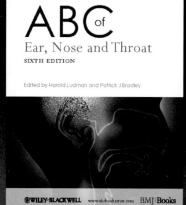

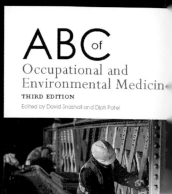

ABC of Pain — Edited by Lesley Colvin and Marie Fallon

ABC of Resuscitation — SIXTH EDITION — Edited by Jasmeet Soar, Gavin D. Perkins and Jerry Nolan

ABC of Ear, Nose and Throat — SIXTH EDITION — Edited by Harold Ludman and Patrick J Bradley

ABC of Occupational and Environmental Medicine — THIRD EDITION — Edited by David Snashall and Dipti Patel

The *ABC* series contains a wealth of indispensable resources for GPs, GP registrars, junior doctors, doctors in training and all those in primary care

▶ **Highly illustrated, informative and a practical source of knowledge**

▶ **An easy-to-use resource, covering the symptoms, investigations, treatment and management of conditions presenting in day-to-day practice and patient support**

▶ **Full colour photographs and illustrations aid diagnosis and patient understanding of a condition**

For more information on all books in the *ABC* series, including links to further information, references and links to the latest official guidelines, please visit:

www.abcbookseries.com

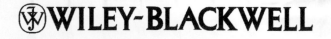

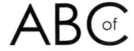

Cancer Care

Carlo Palmieri BSc PhD FRCP

University of Liverpool
The Royal Liverpool University Hospital & The Clatterbridge Cancer Centre
Liverpool, UK

Esther Bird MA MRCP FRCR DFFP

Silverdale GP Surgery
Burgess Hill
West Sussex, UK

Richard Simcock MRCPI FRCR

Sussex Cancer Centre
Brighton and Sussex University Hospitals NHS Trust
Brighton, UK

WILEY-BLACKWELL

A John Wiley & Sons, Ltd., Publication

BMJ|Books

Library of Congress Cataloging-in-Publication Data

ABC of cancer care / edited by Carlo Palmieri, Esther Bird, Richard Simcock.
        p. ; cm.
    Includes bibliographical references and index.
    ISBN 978-0-470-67440-6 (pbk.)
    I. Palmieri, Carlo, 1968– editor of compilation. II. Bird, Esther, 1970– editor of compilation. III. Simcock, Richard, 1969– editor of compilation.
    [DNLM: 1. Neoplasms – therapy. 2. Neoplasms – diagnosis. QZ 266]
    RC261.A7
    616.99'4 – dc23

                                                                    2013008892

A catalogue record for this book is available from the British Library.

Wiley also publishes its books in a variety of electronic formats. Some content that appears in print may not be available in electronic books.

Cover Image used with permission from James Lewis, Clinical Media Centre, Brighton and Sussex University Hospitals NHS Trust. Copyright © 2013, James Lewis & Brighton and Sussex University Hospitals NHS Trust
Cover design by Andy Meanden

Set in 9.25/12 Minion by Laserwords Private Limited, Chennai, India

Printed in Singapore by Ho Printing Singapore Pte Ltd

1 2013

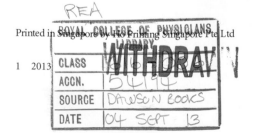

Contents

List of Contributors, vii

Preface, xi

Acknowledgements, xiii

1 Multidisciplinary Care, 1
Richard Simcock

2 Cancer Imaging, 5
Guy Burkill and Adrian K.P. Lim

3 Surgery, 10
Daniel Richard Leff and Richard Simcock

4 Surgery for Metastatic Disease, 15
Timothy W.R. Briggs, Elizabeth J. Gillott, Lewis W. Thorne, and Long R. Jiao

5 Chemotherapy, 20
Catherine Harper-Wynne and Catherine M. Kelly

6 Toxicities of Chemotherapy, 26
Sacha Jon Howell, Alison Jones, and Colin R. James

7 Radiotherapy, 30
Alastair Thomson and Mark Beresford

8 Toxicities of Radiotherapy, 34
Russell Burcombe, Jonathan Hicks, and Richard Simcock

9 Endocrine Therapy, 39
Carlo Palmieri, Matthew Flook, and Duncan C. Gilbert

10 Biological and Targeted Therapies, 44
Ruth E. Board, Jennifer W. Pang, Carlo Palmieri, and Suzy Cleator

11 Trials in Cancer Care, 50
Evandro de Azambuja, David Cameron, and Janet E. Brown

12 Oncological Emergencies, 55
Thomas E. Newsom-Davis and Mohammed Rizwanullah

13 Cancer in the Elderly, 61
Alistair Ring and Juliet E. Wright

14 Nutrition, 64
Mhairi Donald

15 Complementary and Alternative Medicine in Cancer Patients, 69
Richard Simcock and Sarah Cavilla

16 Specialist Nursing Care, 74
Clare Sullivan, Beverley Longhurst, Amelia Cook, Elizabeth Bowman, and Jean Rodell

17 Cancer Survivorship, 78
Esther Bird, Amy Guppy, and Carlo Palmieri

Index, 83

List of Contributors

Mark Beresford DM MA BM Bch MRCP FRCR
Consultant Clinical Oncologist & Visiting Senior Lecturer
Royal United Hospital
Bath, UK

Esther Bird MA MRCP FRCR DFFP
Silverdale GP Surgery
Burgess Hill
West Sussex, UK

Ruth E. Board MBChB PhD
Consultant in Medical Oncology
Rosemere Cancer Centre
Royal Preston Hospital
Preston, UK

Elizabeth Bowman
Breast Clinical Nurse Specialist
The Harley Street Clinic (HCA International)
London, UK

Timothy W.R. Briggs MD(Res) MCh(Orth) FRCS
Consultant Orthopaedic Surgeon
Royal National Orthopaedic Hospital
Stanmore, UK

Janet E. Brown MD FRCP
Senior Clinical Lecturer & Honorary Consultant in Medical Oncology
University of Leeds
St James's University Hospital
Leeds, UK

Russell Burcombe MB BS BSc Hons MD FRCP FRCR
Consultant Clinical Oncologist
Kent Oncology Centre
Maidstone Hospital
Maidstone, Kent, UK

Guy Burkill BSc MB BS MA MRCP FRCR
Consultant Radiologist
Brighton and Sussex University Hospitals NHS Trust
Brighton, UK

David Cameron MD FRCP
Professor of Oncology
University of Edinburgh
Edinburgh, UK

Sarah Cavilla
Specialist Registrar in Clinical Oncology
Sussex Cancer Centre
Brighton and Sussex University Hospitals NHS Trust
Brighton, UK

Suzy Cleator BM BCh MRCP FRCR PhD
Consultant Clinical Oncologist & Honorary Senior Lecturer
Imperial College Healthcare NHS Trust
London, UK

Amelia Cook
Breast Clinical Nurse Specialist
The Harley Street Clinic (HCA International)
London, UK

Evandro de Azambuja MD PhD
Medical Director
BrEAST Data Centre
Jules Bordet Institute
Brussels, Belgium

Mhairi Donald BSc RD
Macmillan Consultant Dietician
Sussex Cancer Centre
Brighton and Sussex University Hospitals NHS Trust
Brighton, UK

Matthew Flook MRCP
Specialist Registrar in Medical Oncology
Department of Medical Oncology
Imperial College Healthcare NHS Trust
London, UK

Duncan C. Gilbert MA MRCP FRCR PhD
Consultant Clinical Oncologist & Honorary Clinical Senior Lecturer
Sussex Cancer Centre
Brighton and Sussex University Hospitals NHS Trust
Brighton, UK

Elizabeth J. Gillott BMedSci MBBS MRCS
Research Fellow
Royal National Orthopaedic Hospital
Stanmore, UK

Amy Guppy MD MRCP
Consultant Medical Oncologist
Mount Vernon Cancer Centre & Hillingdon Hospitals NHS Foundation
Trust
Northwood, Herts, UK

Catherine Harper-Wynne MD FRCP
Consultant Medical Oncologist
Kent Oncology Centre
Maidstone Hospital
Barming, Kent, UK

Jonathan Hicks
Consultant Clinical Oncologist
Beatson West of Scotland Cancer Centre
Glasgow, UK

Sacha Jon Howell MRCP PhD
Senior Lecturer & Honorary Consultant in Medical Oncology
University of Manchester, Institute of Cancer Studies
Department of Medical Oncology
The Christie NHS Foundation Trust
Manchester, UK

Colin R. James PhD MB BCH BAO MRCP
Consultant & Honorary Senior Lecturer in Medical Oncology
Belfast Health and Social Care Trust
Department of Oncology
Northern Ireland Cancer Centre
Belfast City Hospital
Belfast, UK

Long R. Jiao MD FRCS
Reader in Surgery
Consultant Hepatobiliary & Pancreatic Surgeon
Department of Surgery and Cancer
Imperial College London
London, UK

Alison Jones MD FRCP
Consultant Medical Oncologist
Royal Free Hospital and University College Hospital
London, UK

Catherine M. Kelly MB BCh BAO BSc MSc MRCPI
Consultant Medical Oncologist
Department of Medical Oncology
Mater Misericordiae University Hospital
Dublin, Ireland

Daniel Richard Leff MBBS PhD FRCS (Gen Surg)
Cancer Research UK Academic Clinical Lecturer in Surgery
Department of Surgery and Cancer
Cancer Research UK Centre
Imperial College London
London, UK

Adrian K.P. Lim MD FRCR
Consultant Radiologist & Reader in Radiology
Department of Imaging
Imperial College Healthcare NHS Trust
London, UK

Beverley Longhurst
Breast Clinical Nurse Specialist
The Harley Street Clinic (HCA International)
London, UK

Thomas E. Newsom-Davis BSc PhD MRCP
Consultant Medical Oncologist
Chelsea and Westminster Healthcare NHS Foundation Trust
London, UK

Carlo Palmieri BSc PhD FRCP
Professor of Translational Oncology & Consultant Medical Oncologist
University of Liverpool
Department of Molecular & Clinical Cancer Medicine
The Royal Liverpool University Hospital & The Clatterbridge Cancer Centre
Liverpool, UK

Jennifer W. Pang BSc MB ChB
Specialist Registrar in Clinical Oncology
Imperial College Healthcare NHS Trust
London, UK

Alistair Ring MA MD MRCP
Senior Lecturer & Honorary Consultant in Medical Oncology
Brighton and Sussex Medical School
Sussex Cancer Centre
Brighton and Sussex University Hospitals NHS Trust
Brighton, UK

Mohammed Rizwanullah MRCP FRCR
Consultant Clinical Oncologist
Beatson West of Scotland Cancer Centre
Glasgow, UK

Jean Rodell
Breast Clinical Nurse Specialist
The Harley Street Clinic (HCA International)
London, UK

Richard Simcock MRCPI FRCR

Consultant Clinical Oncologist

Sussex Cancer Centre

Brighton and Sussex University Hospitals NHS Trust

Brighton, UK

Clare Sullivan

Breast Clinical Nurse Specialist

The Harley Street Clinic (HCA International)

London, UK

Alastair Thomson BM PGCME MRCP FRCR

Consultant Clinical Oncologist

Royal Cornwall Hospital (Sunrise Centre)

Truro, Cornwall, UK

Lewis W. Thorne MB ChB FRCS(Neurosurgery)

Consultant Neurosurgeon

Victor Horsley Department of Neurosurgery

The National Hospital for Neurology and Neurosurgery

London, UK

Juliet E. Wright MB BS MD FRCP

Senior Lecturer & Honorary Consultant Elderly Medicine

Brighton and Sussex Medical School

Department of Elderly Medicine

Brighton, UK

Preface

Every 2 minutes, someone in the UK is diagnosed with cancer. That amounts to over 300 000 cases per year and a lifetime risk of one in three for any given person. 'Cancer' however is a term which encompasses over 200 diseases, with differing presentations and biologies. Many of these cancer types are increasing in incidence. The average GP in England will see seven new cases of cancer per year and will have an increasing number of survivors under their care. For the NHS, providing care and treatment is hugely costly; £5 billion was spent in England in 2007/08, with 4.7 million bed days used by cancer patients annually.

Although the number of cancers is steadily increasing, so too is the pace of innovation in treating the disease. The last decade has seen continued innovation in all areas of cancer care. The oldest form of cancer treatment, surgery, has been enriched by technological developments and advances in aftercare and rehabilitation. The physics-based specialty of radiation has benefited enormously from developments in computer processor power and chemotherapy has been enhanced not only by new agents but also by supportive drugs. Advances in our knowledge regarding cancer biology have enabled the development and introduction of so-called 'targeted therapies' and have set us on the road to a much more personalised approach to cancer treatment.

Much of this innovation is driven by work in clinical trials and is only made possible by attentive care of the patient through advocacy, nursing and good-quality nutritional care, coordinated by multidisciplinary teams (MDTs). In addition, the contribution of charitable bodies, which fund research, support hospices and provide information and support to patients and their families, plays a key role.

The end result of these innovations is that we have more cancer survivors than ever before and attention can now rightly turn to how these patients can rehabilitate and recover fully from their cancer experience; hence the emerging concept of cancer 'survivorship'.

Given the massive impact of this important disease, it is vital to be able to understand the basic principles underpinning the care of a cancer patient, as well as the myriad treatment options. We have produced this book to give the reader a clear idea of current treatment paradigms in modern cancer care. We have discussed principles, but also included sections outlining the common toxicities. Common emergencies and explanations of cancer care structure are included. Furthermore, we emphasise the importance of holistic care delivered in a multidisciplinary approach.

The book has been written within the context of currently available treatments, both explaining their principles and with an eye to emerging possibilities. It is an exciting time to be involved in treating this disease, with more effective therapies in use than ever before, and we hope this book will prove a useful guide.

Carlo Palmieri
Esther Bird
Richard Simcock

Acknowledgements

We would like to acknowledge the patients who agreed to be photographed or have their images used in this book, by doing so they have helped to ensure that this book is as user friendly, accessible and educational as possible. This book has them in mind, and we hope it will ensure a better understanding of cancer care by non-specialists and students, enabling all those who come into contact with cancer patients to be well informed and better placed to understand, help, guide, treat and support all those diagnosed with cancer.

We thank all those who kindly agreed to become involved and gave up some of their precious free time to author chapters. The care of cancer is a multi-disciplinary approach and this book is a shining example of such team work. We are immensely grateful to Jon Peacock Senior Development Editor, for Health Sciences Books at Wiley-Blackwell for his support and guidance during the development and writing of this book. We also would like to thank Tim West, the Copy-Editor for the book and Neeta Roy, Project Manager at Laserwords and Natra Aziz, Assistant Production Editor at Wiley-Blackwell and their colleagues who help craft the various word documents, pictures and images into the final pages of print which you now see within these covers.

Finally, we are grateful to our parents and families for their love and support as ever.

Carlo Palmieri
Esther Bird
Richard Simcock

CHAPTER 1

Multidisciplinary Care

Richard Simcock

Sussex Cancer Centre, Royal Sussex County Hospital, Brighton, UK

OVERVIEW

- The multidisciplinary team (MDT) has become a vital part of the cancer patient's management
- The multidisciplinary team meeting (MDTM) should lead to improved decision making for the benefit of the patient
- Multidisciplinary teams will be constituted differently according to the cancer type
- Decisions on cancer treatment intent and modality depend on the cancer stage and patient performance status and fitness
- The MDTM allows for review of pathology and histology specimens in the diagnosis of the patient's cancer
- Cancer waiting time targets have increased the speed at which patients are treated for cancer in the UK

Introduction

Cancer care is complex. The first treatments were either palliation or surgery. During the twentieth century nonsurgical oncology grew exponentially to provide radiotherapy and chemotherapy. In this century we have begun to see an explosion in biological and targeted therapies, as well as technical developments in the delivery of surgery and radiation. This has been accompanied by parallel improvements in imaging and pathology, and an increasing recognition of the roles of advocacy, support and survivorship. In order to deliver best care for a cancer patient, it has become necessary to form teams to provide all the requisite expertise.

Before the early 1990s, only a small proportion of cancer patients benefited from their care being managed by a team of cancer specialists, meaning that care was often not specialist and that staff worked in isolation. Data collection was poor, as was communication between primary and secondary care.

In 1995, the Calman–Hine report recommended a reorganisation of cancer services such that whenever possible, cancer was managed by a multidisciplinary team (MDT). The MDT is defined in the Department of Health (DH)'s *Manual for Cancer Services* as the meeting of a group of professionals at a given time or place to make decisions regarding treatment options for individual patients. In 2000, Cancer Networks were formed to bring together the providers of cancer care (organisations that deliver cancer services to patients) and the commissioners of cancer care (organisations that plan, purchase and monitor cancer services) in order that they could work together to plan and deliver high-quality cancer services for specific populations. There are currently 28 Cancer Networks in England.

Since 1995, the establishment of MDTs in the UK has been mandated by the requirements of peer review, a process led by the National Cancer Action Team and monitored by Networks. Over 95% cancers are now managed by an MDT.

Common cancers (e.g. breast and lung) are often managed by MDTs based at the local hospital. Rarer cancers (e.g. head and neck) may be referred to a Network specialist MDT based at the cancer centre within the Network. Very rare cancers (e.g. sarcoma) may be managed by a regional MDT serving several Cancer Networks.

The MDT will usually meet on a regular basis to discuss cases at a multidisciplinary team meeting (MDTM). The MDTM requires careful preparation and review of clinical materials before discussion by the wider team. Frequently, members from the wider team will use teleconferencing facilities to join discussions. Supporting a large team and investing in required the infrastructure is expensive; cost estimates range from approximately £90 per patient discussion in a high-volume local breast MDTM to more than double that for a regional specialist head and neck MDTM.

Membership of the MDT is determined by the needs of patients and will vary according to the disease. The MDT is made up of clerical and support staff, core members whose presence is essential to decision making and extended members who will have valuable input into the processes of the MDT and into occasional individual patients. Core members are expected to attend each MDTM (see Table 1.1).

Evidence for MDT working

It has proved difficult to gain evidence for the effectiveness of MDTs due to their universal implementation (preventing control groups) and the concurrent changes in cancer treatment (complicating historical comparisons). Nonetheless, there are data which show improvements in cancer outcomes, including survival, in areas which implemented MDT processes compared to areas which did

ABC of Cancer Care, First Edition.
Edited by Carlo Palmieri, Esther Bird and Richard Simcock.
© 2013 John Wiley & Sons, Ltd. Published 2013 by John Wiley & Sons, Ltd.

Table 1.1 Core and extended members for breast and head and neck cancer MDTs. MDTs will be constituted differently according to the expertise required to give best care for each type of cancer.

	Breast MDT	Head and neck MDT
Common core members	Team secretary MDT coordinator Clinical nurse specialist Pathologist Radiologist Oncologist	
Core members	Breast surgeon	ENT surgeons Maxillofacial surgeons Plastic surgeons Restorative dentist Speech and language therapist Senior ward nurse Palliative care specialist Dietitian
Common extended members	Social worker Psychiatrist/clinical psychologist Physiotherapist Occupational therapist	
Extended members	GP Palliative care specialist Breast radiographer Plastic surgeon Clinical geneticist/genetics counsellor Lymphoedema specialist Orthopaedic surgeon with expertise in management of bone metastases Neurosurgeon	Anaesthetist with a special interest in head and neck cancer Gastroenterologist Ophthalmologist Pain management specialist Nuclear medicine specialist Therapeutic radiographer Maxillofacial/dental technician Dental hygienist

not. A large retrospective cohort study of nearly 14 000 patients in neighbouring areas in Scotland showed 18% lower breast cancer mortality in the area introducing MDTs (despite a higher mortality prior to MDT working).

MDT working also appears to increase work-related satisfaction in the team, as well as clinical trial recruitment.

Having a broader range of professional opinions available seems likely to benefit a patient. Teams are likely to generate higher-quality solutions and to have a wider sense of 'ownership' of the eventual decision. There are however problems inherent in the team decision-making process: it may dominated by individuals, or the team may be susceptible to 'groupthink' (defined as a deterioration in mental efficiency and moral judgement as a result of in-group pressure). Psychologists have also described 'risky shift', in which the decision made carries higher risk than that made by individuals, as the group feels reduced accountability.

A survey of over 2000 MDT members conducted by the National Cancer Action Team in the UK concluded that the most important aspects of MDT effectiveness were leadership, communication between members and time for preparation.

Databases

The MDT is the perfect forum in which to capture detailed disease data. These give epidemiological data and highlight regional and local variations in disease presentation and treatments. Many MDTs will use purpose-built data information systems such as the Somerset data system (developed by health care staff in Somerset) and commercial systems (e.g. InfoFlex).

In addition to these local databases, MDTs in England are mandated to supply information to various national cancer audits, including LUCADA (for lung cancer), DAHNO (for head and neck cancer) and the National Colorectal Audit.

Cancer waiting times

Patients may be referred directly to an MDT by primary care doctors who suspect cancer. Facilitating this process, there are agreed key symptoms/signs listed on referral pro formas in order to help triage (see Table 1.2). Patients referred to secondary care and subsequently found to have cancer should be 'fast tracked' into the MDT. Patients may also enter the MDT system as a result of participation in national screening programs for breast, colorectal and cervical cancers.

In 2000, the NHS introduced cancer waiting times which specified that patients with suspected breast cancer should be seen within 2 weeks of referral. These waiting times have been expanded such that in 2011 there is now a comprehensive set for all cancers (see Figure 1.1). An MDT has an administrator (sometimes referred to as a 'patient pathway coordinator') who tracks and reports these wait times nationally. Studies of MDTs show that they reduce cancer wait times.

In the UK, over 95% of people are now seen by a specialist within 2 weeks of an urgent GP referral for suspected cancer and over 98% of people treated receive their first definitive treatment within 31 days of receiving their diagnosis.

Treatment intent

A fundamental principle of treatment selection is deciding the intent of treatment. The MDT will use information on staging and patient

Table 1.2 Examples of referral pro formas used in primary care, detailing symptoms that may lead to suspicion of cancer (lung and upper gastrointestinal (GI) cancer shown).

Lung	Upper GI
Persistent haemoptysis in smoker or ex-smoker >40 years	Dysphagia
Unexplained or persistent symptoms (>3 weeks):	Persistent vomiting and weight loss
• cough	Unexplained iron-deficiency anaemia
• wheeze	Unexplained weight loss
• weight loss	Unexplained abdominal pain and weight loss
Breathlessness	Upper abdominal mass
Chest/shoulder pain	Obstructive jaundice

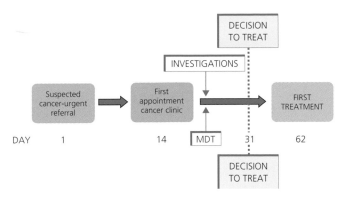

CANCER WAITING TIMES–NATIONAL STANDARDS, UK

Figure 1.1 National cancer waiting times and the cancer care pathway. Updated version of the national cancer waiting times originally set out in the NHS Cancer Action Plan (2000). There are three national cancer waiting time standards designed to reduce waiting times between referral and diagnosis and between diagnosis and treatment: (1) 2-week wait rule – all patients with an urgent GP referral for suspected cancer should wait not more than 14 days between referral (Day 1) and assessment by a hospital specialist (Day 14); (2) 62-day standard – all patients referred under the 2-week wait rule should be assessed and have treatment initiated within 62 days; (3) 31-day standard – cancer patients should wait no more than 31 days to receive their treatment from the date the treatment decision is made, regardless of their referral priority. The initial MDTM discussion (and necessary investigations) usually takes place between the patient's first assessment in clinic and the date their treatment decision is made. However, there is no mandatory date for the MDTM.

fitness to determine whether treatment will be radical (aimed at cancer cure) or palliative (aimed at symptom control and/or life extension). 'Adjuvant therapy' is a term derived from the Latin *adjuvans*, 'to help', and describes treatment given as an addition to radical therapy. Neoadjuvant treatment (usually chemotherapy) is given before planned radical therapy.

There are multiple factors which influence treatment selection (see Box 1.1).

Box 1.1 **Factors influencing treatment selection by the MDT**

- Age.
- Stage/extent of disease.
- Prognosis.
- Functional status.
- Comorbidities/general health.
- Performance score.
- Previous treatments.
- Whether primary is known.
- Magnitude of treatment (e.g. intensive long-course chemotherapy or difficult surgery).
- Fitness for surgery/anaesthesia.
- Likelihood of complications.
- Ability to rehabilitate after treatment.

Staging

The MDT will use review of radiological imaging (see Chapter 2) to help establish the disease stage using an agreed staging system

(Tumour/Node/Metastasis (TNM) or American Joint Committee on Cancer (AJCC)). The MDT radiologist will have organ-specific imaging expertise and will be able to direct the most appropriate imaging sequence. The team will also have a histopathologist as a key core member, who will review biopsy and excision specimens, the pathology being crucial to the correct diagnosis. As with radiology, the pathologist will have disease-specific expertise and will be able to guide specialist immunohistochemistry to assist diagnosis. Increasingly, the specialist MDT pathologist will be involved after diagnosis in establishing whether specific molecular markers of treatment sensitivity are present (e.g. HER-2 status in breast cancer, KRAS mutations in colorectal cancer, BRAF mutation in melanoma). After diagnosis and following radical surgery, the pathologist will liaise with the operating surgical team at the MDTM to review the excised disease and establish risks for recurrence in order to assist the oncologists in planning adjuvant treatments.

Patient assessments

Along with the correct diagnosis and staging of the disease, an accurate assessment of the patient's fitness is required. The most useful and simple patient assessment is the performance status score. The Karnofsky (Table 1.3) and the ECOG/WHO/Zubrod (Table 1.4) scores are 10- and 5-point systems respectively which summarise a patient's global health and ability. The ECOG/WHO/Zubrod score was developed in 1982. Despite its simplicity, it has very high predictive and prognostic value in evaluating a patient's likely response in almost all cancers. It is good practice to record the performance score of each patient.

More complex patient assessment tools are available, particularly for the elderly cancer patient (see Chapter 13).

What makes an effective MDT

An MDT makes treatment recommendations rather than decisions (which require dialogue with the patient). An effective MDT will do this best when membership consists of the correct specialists and there is appropriate time to prepare. The effective

Table 1.3 Karnofsky Performance Status score.

Rating	Meaning
100%	Normal, no complaints, no signs of disease
90%	Capable of normal activity, few symptoms or signs of disease
80%	Normal activity with some difficulty, some symptoms or signs
70%	Caring for self, not capable of normal activity or work
60%	Requiring some help, can take care of most personal requirements
50%	Requires help often, requires frequent medical care
40%	Disabled, requires special care and help
30%	Severely disabled, hospital admission indicated but no risk of death
20%	Very ill, urgently requiring admission, requires supportive measures or treatment
10%	Moribund, rapidly progressive fatal disease processes
0%	Death

Table 1.4 ECOG/WHO/Zubrod performance status score.

Grade	Meaning
0	Fully active, able to carry on all pre-disease performance without restriction
1	Restricted in physically strenuous activity but ambulatory and able to carry out work of a light or sedentary nature, e.g. light house work, office work
2	Ambulatory and capable of self-care but unable to carry out any work activities, up and about more than 50% of waking hours
3	Capable of only limited self-care, confined to bed or chair more than 50% of waking hours
4	Completely disabled, cannot carry out any self-care, totally confined to bed or chair
5	Dead

MDT will communicate well with its members but also with primary and secondary care. Adherence to guidance should be high, as should recruitment to clinical trials. Improved outcomes for the patient and better satisfaction for the staff should be the outcome.

Further reading

National Cancer Action Team (n.d.) Ensuring better treatment: multi-disciplinary team development, http://ncat.nhs.uk/our-work/ensuring-better-treatment/multi-disciplinary-team-development# (last accessed 8 March 2013).

National Cancer Action Team (2010) Characteristics of an effective multi-disciplinary team (MDT), http://ncat.nhs.uk/sites/default/files/work-docs/NCATMDTCharacteristics.pdf (last accessed 8 March 2013).

National Health Service (2011) *National Cancer Peer Review Programme Handbook*, available from http://www.cquins.nhs.uk/?menu=about-us-background (last accessed 8 March 2013).

National Institute for Clinical Excellence (n.d.) NICE guidance, http://guidance.nice.org.uk/ (last accessed 8 March 2013).

CHAPTER 2

Cancer Imaging

Guy Burkill[1] and Adrian K.P. Lim[2]

[1]Brighton and Sussex University Hospitals NHS Trust, Brighton, UK
[2]Imperial College Healthcare NHS Trust, London, UK

OVERVIEW

- Radiology is an essential element of cancer care in staging, and increasingly in response assessment and interventional treatments
- Accurate radiological staging may prevent futile treatments and guide treatment selection
- Different modalities offer different sensitivies for imaging of tumours, regional nodes and metastases
- Technological advancements are improving the sensitivies of all modalities
- Nuclear medicine and functional MRI give information about the biological properties of tissue, in addition to anatomical data

---

Introduction

The past 40 years have witnessed an explosion in medical imaging. It now impacts on all cancer patients at many points on their pathway. Traditionally used to guide diagnosis and staging and determine treatment response, it is now also used to deliver treatments with both palliative and curative intent. This growth in imaging offers many tests – often more than one for the same indication. Preferred tests are influenced by competing factors, including accuracy, cost and availability (Table 2.1).

The risks of radiation exposure are also important. Medical/dental imaging now accounts for 90% of all artificial radiation. Estimates suggest that 1.5–2.0% of cancers in the USA may be attributable to computed tomography (CT). Although in cancer patients the individual risk may be commuted by limited prognosis, greater consideration should be afforded to children, given their longer life expectancy and increased sensitivity to radiation (2–5 times that of adults).

Useful guidance when deciding which test to choose has recently been updated by both UK and US radiology colleges (see Further Reading).

ABC of Cancer Care, First Edition.
Edited by Carlo Palmieri, Esther Bird and Richard Simcock.
© 2013 John Wiley & Sons, Ltd. Published 2013 by John Wiley & Sons, Ltd.

TNM staging

Staging is the process of determining the location and extent of a malignant disease. Now in its seventh edition (2010), the American Joint Committee on Cancer (AJCC) sets out through an evidence-based review of impacts on survival how clinicians, radiologists and pathologists stage cancers with regard to the primary tumour (T), lymph nodes (N) and distant metastases (M). Imaging tests typically perform best at one or two of these subsections, but not all three; hence the frequent need for multiple staging investigations.

Plain film

Plain-film radiography in cancer care has largely been usurped by other modalities. The most common cancer indications include first detection of lung and bone tumours and the investigation of symptoms during treatment or follow up (e.g. neutropenic sepsis and drug related lung injury (see Chapter 6)). Chest x-ray (CXR) is a relatively insensitive and nonspecific test that has been repeatedly investigated as a screening tool for lung cancer but not shown to be effective (see Figure 2.1). However, plain radiographs are normally the initial investigation of choice due to their low cost and wide availability.

Fluoroscopy

Fluoroscopy uses x-rays in real time rather than as a still image. It now uses sophisticated devices deployed by interventional radiologists to guide stent placement, in order to relieve malignant obstructions of the bowel, bile duct and veins, as well as to deliver targeted therapy such as radioactive microspheres to liver tumours. In addition, it is used for the placing of lines or ports, enabling delivery of systemic treatment (see Chapter 5).

Mammography

Mammography remains the imaging of choice for breast screening in the UK. It is better at detecting microcalcification (MCC) than are ultrasound and magnetic resonance imaging (MRI), which are superior in assessing the density of a breast lesion and, in the case of MRI, enhancement characteristics.

Mammography uses conventional x-rays but is moving to digital use rather than x-ray film. In digital mammography, conventional

Table 2.1 Overview of imaging tests in oncology.

Modality	Dose	Cost	Comment
Plain film	☢	£	First detection for lung and bone tumours Typically insensitive and nonspecific Further imaging usually required
Mammography	☢☢☢	£	Used in national screening programme Always consists of two views Radiological investigation of choice for initial imaging of most breast problems
Ultrasound	None	££	Widely available Often an early test in the patient pathway. Particularly used in the diagnosis of breast, gynaecological and testicular malignancy Best modality for image-guided tissue biopsy and drainage Limited by gas in bowel and lung
CT	☢☢☢☢☢	£££	Most versatile all-round modality in cancer imaging Typically the next test after plain film and ultrasound Drawbacks include radiation dose and poor accuracy for lymph node staging Gatekeeper to PET-CT for many tumours
MRI	None	££££	Test of choice for primary tumour staging of bone, most head and neck, male and female pelvic and anorectal cancers Superior to CT for lymph node staging and liver lesion characterisation Test of choice for suspected cord compression Considerably slower than CT
PET-CT	☢☢☢☢☢☢☢	£££££	Still limited availability Best test for detecting metastases in most cancers and so changing treatment intent Glucose uptake not specific and insufficient in low-grade tumours False-positive glucose uptake by infection/inflammation can be a problem Will require development of further tracers for greater specificity and earlier cancer detection

CT, computed tomography; PET-CT, positron emission tomography – computed tomography; MRI, magnetic resonance imaging. Radiation effective doses for a chest x-ray are in the range of 0.014 mSV (millisiverts), mammography 0.3 mSv, CT of chest abdomen and pelvis 10 mSv and whole-body PET-CT 14 mSv (from Hart *et al.* 2008).

film is replaced with solid-state detectors that convert x-rays into electrical signals, which then produce computer-generated images of the breast.

The move from analogue to digital has improved the spatial resolution of mammography and has allowed tomograms of the breast (similar to CT), a technology known as tomosynthesis. This latest technique is yet to find regular clinical application but early studies suggest that it allows composite shadowing to be clearly distinguished from a mass or distortion with greater confidence. It does not, however, improve on the detection or characterisation of MCC, where mammography remains superior. While mammography is better for detecting MCC and therefore ductal carcinoma in situ (DCIS), tumour extent is better delineated with MRI, where tissue enhancement is key.

Ultrasound

Diagnostic ultrasound utilises probes of frequencies varying between 2 and 18 mHz. These probes act as transmitters and receivers of the returning sound waves in order to generate an image. In general, the higher the frequency, the better the resolution but the poorer the penetration. The converse is also true.

Ultrasound is particularly good for assessing the solid organs, especially the liver, where it plays a significant role in staging disease, for example in patients with breast cancer, or as surveillance in detecting primary liver tumours in patients with chronic liver disease, as well as determining indeterminate low density lesions detected on a staging CT. It is very good at distinguishing solid

from fluid-filled lesions and has fine resolution; lesions only a few millimetres in diameter can be outlined clearly. Ultrasound is limited by body habitus, where large patients reduce the penetration of the sound waves and thus image resolution.

Endoscopic ultrasound (EUS), where an ultrasound probe is attached to an endoscope, has proved invaluable in assessing structures in the chest (endobronchial ultrasound, EBUS) and abdomen, which can be obscured by gas; as the lesions are closer to the probe, it also offers significantly better resolution. It helps with assessing the bowel or airway wall, pancreatic/retroperitoneal lesions and lymph nodes. Another advantage is that lesions can be sampled at time of examination.

The advent of microbubbles, a contrast agent for ultrasound, has significantly improved the sensitivity and specificity for the detection and characterisation of focal liver lesions, so that they rival those of CT and MRI. In particular, contrast-enhanced ultrasound has a very high sensitivity in the detection of metastases where they appear as defects in the late phase; that is, past the portal phase of enhancement at around 2–3 minutes post injection. Lesions as small as 3–5 mm can be accurately characterised.

Owing to its wide availability, ultrasound remains the initial imaging modality when it comes to assessing the solid organs in the abdomen. Its easy manouvrebility and good spatial resolution, particularly with superficial and small structures, also make it the modality of choice for the assessment of palpable 'lumps and bumps'. It is the most utilised modality for image guided biopsy.

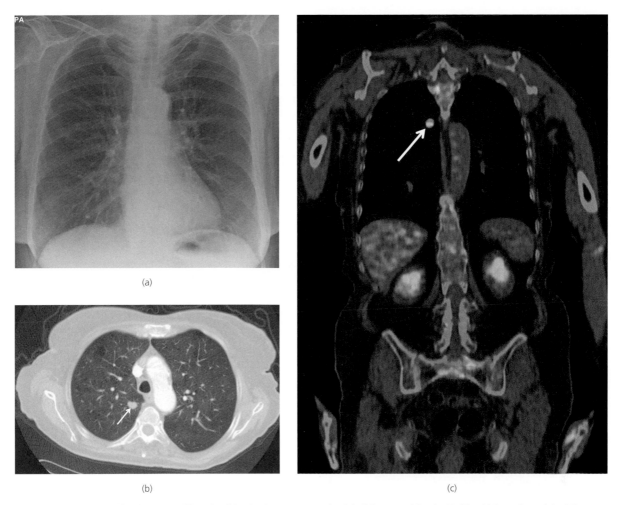

(a)

(b)

(c)

Figure 2.1 CXR (a) was requested for shortness of breath. This raised concern over the right hilum, resulting in CT (b), which confirmed the hilum as normal but revealed a CXR occult lung carcinoma (arrow). PET-CT (c) showed stage T1aN0M0 (arrow), so this was treated with curative resection.

Computed tomography

CT is the foundation test for many cancer patients. The majority of cancers are staged with CT and it is the most common imaging test for radiotherapy treatment planning, response assessment, surveillance (when appropriate) and suspected relapse. It provides an excellent overview of disease in an economical (NHS tariff for body CT = £144), readily available and rapid test (a whole-body CT takes just seconds to acquire). It also acts as a 'gatekeeper' to more costly, less available complimentary modalities; for example, in oesophageal cancer staging it provides an overview of disease extent. If CT reveals no distant disease, EUS is used for more accurate primary (T) and lymph node (N) staging and positron emission tomography – computed tomography (PET-CT) as a more sensitive search for metastases (M). Where greater tissue contrast is required to separate tumour from normal structures, MRI outperforms CT; for example, in the staging of rectal, uterine and cervix cancers. An emerging role for CT is cancer screening. The bowel cancer screening programme uses CT colonography when colonoscopy is unacceptable or incomplete. The National Lung Screening Trial (NLST) was stopped prematurely after it revealed that low-dose CT screening of high-risk individuals reduced disease specific mortality by 20%. The results of a UK trial are awaited and a cost–benefit analysis is required before it is adopted by the NHS.

Magnetic resonance imaging

MRI technology is advancing, with larger field strength magnets providing improved image quality, particularly with 3 Tesla (T) MRI scanners. The majority of clinical scanners at present work at 1.5 T. MRI is absolutely contraindicated in patients with pacemakers and there is still concern regarding the safety of scanning patients with metalwork at higher field strengths.

MRI provides very good soft tissue differentiation when compared to CT or ultrasound but is hampered by relatively long scanning times and therefore movement artefacts. Scan times are getting progressively faster, with stronger gradients and advancing technology.

Altering sequences and tissue weightings can help better evaluate different types of tissue and advancing techniques such as diffusion weighted imaging (DWI) and magnetic resonance spectroscopy (MRS) can provide an insight into the metabolic activity of lesions. The restriction of water mobility within a cellular environment in DWI is thought to represent an early harbinger of biological abnormality. These additional DWI sequences may be useful in assessing the aggressiveness of lesions and in tumour response. MRS, on the other hand, gives information on chemical cellular content where graphs are obtained. The graph profiles of malignant and benign tissues will differ due to their contrasting tissue compositions. This currently remains a research technique.

As with the other cross-sectional imaging techniques, contrast enhancement with intravenous gadolinium-based agents can help improve tissue differentiation and assess the vascularity of lesions. There are also contrast agents with a reticulendothelial uptake phase and some which are biliary excreted; therefore, the examination can be tailored to suit the organ or clinical scenario of choice.

In cancer imaging, MRI is not yet typically used for whole-body staging; this is partly due to cost, but it also has limited accuracy in lung lesions when compared with CT. Typically, MRI is used to assess locoregional spread and stage of disease. For example, in colorectal, prostate or gynaecological cancers, MRI provides highly accurate tumour extent and lymph node staging.

MRI has proved invaluable at imaging the central nervous system (CNS) and spine for malignancy and particularly cord compression, where it remains the modality of choice over the other cross-sectional techniques.

Overall, this field continues to advance rapidly, and whole-body MRI is now possible. In some instances it has been used as a screening tool or in the detection of metastases and disease response, but its clinical value and efficacy in this respect remain a subject of study.

Nuclear medicine

Nuclear medicine studies function at a molecular level rather than through changes in anatomy. There are a plethora of tests, which rely on increasingly specific radiopharmaceuticals to image or treat cancer patients. Gamma and PET cameras have relatively

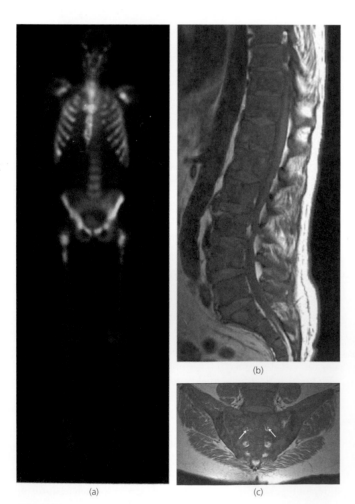

Figure 2.2 Prostate cancer with disseminated bone metastases on bone scan (a). Later presentation with sacral nerve root signs. MRI (b,c) revealed both the extensive bone marrow infiltration and the sacral foraminal narrowing (arrow).

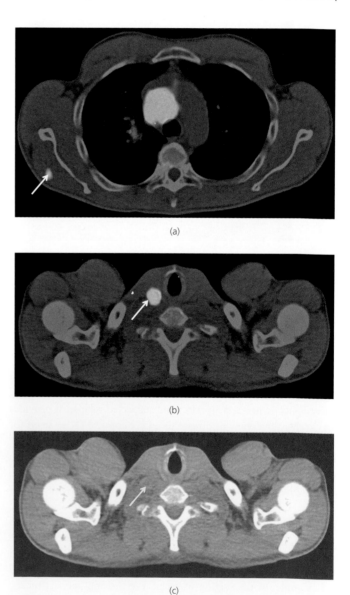

Figure 2.3 PET-CT (a,b) staging for lung cancer. The large CT-evident mediastinal lymph node (N2) was intensely FDG avid. PET also revealed an avid supraclavicular fossa lymph node (N3) (arrow) not apparent on CT (c), even in hindsight, as well as an intramuscular metastasis (arrow) also occult on CT. Stage migration between tests was T2aN2M0 to T2aN3M1b.

Lung

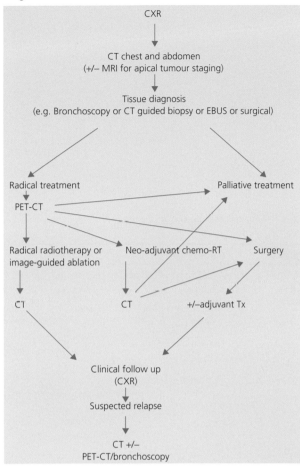

Rectal

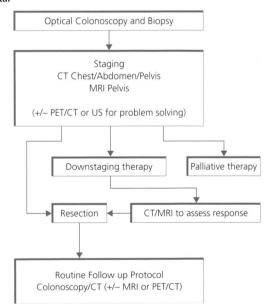

Figure 2.4 Algorithm of typical patient pathways for lung and colorectal cancer, illustrating where imaging may be used and the preferred imaging modality.

poor image resolution, so are increasingly combined with CT and more recently MRI scanners to create fused functional and anatomical data. Despite the unique potential for individually tailored imaging agents, the majority of nuclear medicine tests performed in cancer patients are technetium 99m bone scans for the detection of metastases and ^{18}F-FDG PET-CT, which observes nonspecific glucose uptake by highly metabolic cancer cells.

Bone scanning relies on osteoblastic activity, so is most accurate when searching for sclerotic bone metastases, from the prostate and breast, for example (see Figure 2.2). False positives may occur when scanning patients in the recovery phase of treatments, whereby healing tissue may be mistaken for active disease. MRI and PET-CT are superior to bone scanning where lesions are lytic, such as in renal cell cancer. MRI is used in preference to the other modalities where spinal cord/nerve compression is suspected (see Chapter 12).

PET-CT infrequently improves T-staging over CT or MRI and, while better for N-staging (CT N-staging in lung cancer: sensitivity 51%, specificity 86%), remains insufficiently accurate to determine management alone (10% false-negative rate in lung cancer), ensuring a role for mediastinal sampling in presurgical staging. Where PET-CT outperforms other tests is in metastatic detection. Among patients staged by CT, PET-CT prevents futile thoracotomy in 20% (Figure 2.3).

To gain some understanding of how these tests interleave in a patient's cancer journey, two typical pathways are outlined in Figure 2.4.

Further reading

American College of Radiology (2011) ACR appropriateness criteria, available from http://www.acr.org/ (last accessed 8 March 2013).

Brenner, D.J. & Hall, E.J. (2007) Computed tomography – an increasing source of radiation exposure. *New England Journal of Medicine*, **357**, 2277–2284.

Edge, S.B., Byrd, D.R., Compton, C.C., Fritz, A.G., Greene, F.L. & Trotti, A. (2010) *AJCC Cancer Staging Manual*, 7th edn. Springer, New York.

Hart, D., Wall, B.F., Hillier, M.C. & Shrimpton, P.C. (2008) Frequency and collective dose for medical and dental x-ray examinations in the UK, 2008. HPA-CRCE-012, http://www.hpa.org.uk/webc/HPAwebFile/HPAweb_C/1287148001641 (last accessed 8 March 2013).

Medina, L.S., Blackmore, C.C. & Applegate, K.E. (2011) *Evidence Based Imaging*. Springer, New York.

The Royal College of Radiologists (2011). iRefer (2011) – making the best use of clinical radiology, available from http://www.rcr.ac.uk/ (last accessed 8 March 2013).

CHAPTER 3

Surgery

Daniel Richard Leff[1] *and Richard Simcock*[2]

[1]Cancer Research UK Centre, Imperial College London, London, UK
[2]Sussex Cancer Centre, Royal Sussex County Hospital, Brighton, UK

OVERVIEW

- Oncological surgery aims to remove an entire tumour with a clear margin of healthy tissue. Acceptable margin distance varies between cancer types
- Preoperative staging is essential, but modalities vary between disease types and according to patterns of disease spread
- Operative techniques have been improved by technological developments such as sentinel node localisation, robotic surgery and navigation systems
- Plastic surgery reconstruction techniques have massively improved cosmetic and functional outcomes from surgery
- Enhanced recovery programmes shorten patients' hospital stays and convalescence

---

Principles

Surgery is the most long established of all cancer treatments, with descriptions of cancer surgery recorded in Egyptian hieroglyphs. Technologies for staging, preoperative preparation, operation, reconstruction and rehabilitation are all continually being developed.

Staging

Developments in imaging and multidisciplinary team (MDT) review (see Chapters 1 and 2) have allowed surgical teams to more comprehensively stage a disease and assess fitness before attempting surgery. This can help to avoid futile surgery, guide surgical decision making and plan reconstruction (see Table 3.1).

Radiological advances must be combined with clinical skill. In rectal cancer, clinical examination enables assessment of fixity to local structures (e.g. vagina) and provides important clues as to the distance from the anal sphincter complex, determining whether a continence-preserving procedure is feasible.

Table 3.1 Elements and modalities of preoperative staging according to disease type.

Staging	Purpose	Examples
Fully stage the disease prior to radical surgery	To detect advanced nodal disease	PET scanning in lung cancer
	To detect metastatic disease	CT scanning of chest and abdomen in upper GI cancer
		Bone scanning in prostate cancer
	To exclude synchronous disease	CT scanning of lungs in head and neck cancer
		Colonoscopy/CT colonography in colorectal cancer
Assess tumour size and position	To determine whether organ preservation is possible	Mammography/MRI in breast cancer
		MRI scanning in head and neck cancer
	To determine the extent of surgery	Ultrasound of axilla in breast cancer
	To determine the functional impact of surgery	MRI and digital examination in rectal cancer
	To plan the operative approach	MRI fusion and navigation systems in brain tumours
	To plan reconstruction	MRI angiography of vessels leading to tissue flaps used for reconstruction

PET, positron emission tomography; CT, computed tompography; GI, gastrointestinal; MRI, magnetic resonance imaging.

Preoperative therapy

The MDT will assess staging information and in some cases recommend other therapies as adjunct to surgery. Preoperative therapy may be chemotherapy (e.g. in breast or oesophageal cancer) or radiotherapy (e.g. in rectal cancer). Surgery may be planned to be followed by further treatments. Breast-conserving surgery, for example, has been able to replace mastectomy in many cases due to the extra local control afforded by postoperative radiotherapy.

ABC of Cancer Care, First Edition.
Edited by Carlo Palmieri, Esther Bird and Richard Simcock.
© 2013 John Wiley & Sons, Ltd. Published 2013 by John Wiley & Sons, Ltd.

Close liaison between members of the MDT is required to plan these sequences of therapy.

Preoperative preparation

Prior to surgery, patients should be carefully consented for treatment. In addition to being made to understand the role and practicalities of surgery, patients need to be guided through functional outcomes. In bowel or urological surgery, the need for a stoma must be carefully discussed with the patient and a stoma nurse specialist should see the patient to mark the ideal site, discuss appliances and provide reassurance and support. In head and neck cancer, a speech and language therapist should counsel the patient on voice and swallow outcomes, while a breast care nurse should assist a breast patient facing choices around reconstruction (see Chapter 16).

Surgery is a major physiological stress. Increasingly there is a focus on optimising the patient's condition perioperatively. Such 'enhanced recovery programmes' (ERPs) are designed to speed patient recovery following major surgery. ERPs are most advanced in bowel and pelvic surgery. In colorectal surgery there is no evidence that bowel preparation improves outcomes, so many surgeons omit purgatives. Carbohydrate drinks and immunonutritients taken just prior to surgery have been shown to improve clinical outcomes following major gastrointestinal (GI) resections and are given in the preoperative period.

Prophylactic antibiotics reduce the risk of infection and should be administered on induction in bowel surgery. Cancer patients are a high-risk group for venous thromboembolism, and thromboprophylaxis in the form of prophylactic low-molecular-weight heparin should be prescribed.

Intraoperative staging

The patient's disease may be further staged during the operation in order to limit the surgical extent and reduce postoperative complications. An example is sentinel lymph node biopsy (SLNB) in breast cancer.

Axillary metastatic disease in breast cancer is a powerful predictor of prognosis, and accurate staging is critical. Traditionally, the axilla was staged by a complete dissection of the axillary fat, fascia and nodes, with the consequent problems of lymphoedema, seroma formation and shoulder restriction. SLNB is now the standard of care. The sentinel node represents the first axillary node-draining breast lymph and is localised preoperatively using injection of a blue dye into periaerolar tissues just prior to the procedure and injection of radioisotope-labelled albumin in the breast. These markers pass to the first draining lymph nodes and are localised visually by the presence of blue dye and the detection of radioactivity using a hand held gamma probe (see Figure 3.1). This 'dual localisation' technique has a 98% success rate for sentinel node identification. When the node is clear of disease, further axillary surgery can be avoided, while a positive node leads to a clearance, in which all the nodes medial to pectoralis minor are removed. Completion axillary clearance is commonly conducted at a second operative procedure; however, the excised node can be sent for immediate frozen section histological analysis or touch imprint cytology, in which a divided node is touched on to a slide for cytological analysis. Automated methods of molecular quantification (one-step nucleic acid amplification, OSNA) facilitate 'live' intraoperative decisions regarding the need to proceed to clearance. SLNB is associated with reduced lymphoedema,

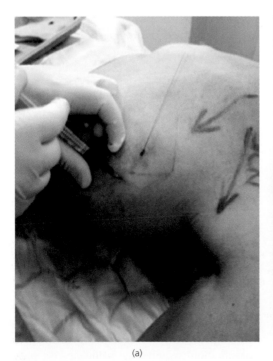
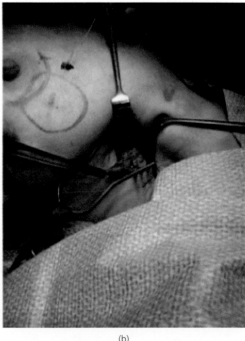

(a)   (b)

Figure 3.1 (a) Patent Blue dye is injected around the tumour at the time of surgery. Note that this patient has had her tumour localised by a guide wire placed in the centre of the tumour by radiologists prior to the operation. (b) When the axilla is dissected, the sentinel node can be identified and removed, having taken up blue dye (see centre of image).

shoulder restriction and enhanced quality of life compared to axillary clearance.

Sentinel node procedures are also utilised in melanoma surgery.

Operative approach

The degree of surgery will vary according to the case. There is an agreed nomenclature that may define different versions of the same operation (Table 3.2).

Technical developments

Computer-assisted surgery

Modern imaging data can now made be available to the operating surgeon in real time. Computer-assisted surgery (CAS) or

Table 3.2 Differences between two types of common cancer surgery.

Mastectomy in breast cancer	Neck dissection in head and neck cancer
Radical Halstead mastectomy: involves removal of the breast gland, axillary tissue and pectoralis muscle. No longer used, as this aggressive approach does not improve survival	*Radical neck dissection*: all ipsilateral lymph nodes from level I to V are removed along with the spinal accessory nerve, internal jugular vein and sternocleinomastoid muscle
Simple mastectomy: removal of the breast gland without any dissection of the axilla	*Modified radical neck dissection*: as for radical neck dissection, with preservation of one or more nonlymphatic structure. Sometimes referred to as a 'functional' neck dissection
Skin sparing mastectomy: facilitates removal of the breast while simultaneously preserving as much of the native skin envelope as possible in order to maximise cosmesis following immediate breast reconstruction	*Selective neck dissection*: one or more of the lymphatic groups normally removed in the radical neck dissection is preserved. The lymph node groups removed are based on patterns of metastases, which are predictable for each site of the disease
Patey mastectomy: a modified radical mastectomy often required for locally advanced primary breast cancer. Involves the removal of the entire breast gland, skin overlying the tumour and all of the axillary fat and lymph nodes	*Extended neck dissection*: additional lymph node groups or nonlymphatic structures are removed
Subcutaneous mastectomy: describes approaches that seek to preserve both the overlying skin envelope and the patient's own nipple aerolar complex. Nipple-sparing mastectomy, as it is also known, is occasionally performed in the context of risk reduction for patients with inherited gene defects (e.g. BRCA 1, BRCA 2) who wish to reduce their risk of breast cancer while maximising their cosmetic outcome	

navigation surgery can 'map' these imaging data to the patient's external anatomy and display the result in theatre on screens. Feedback from special surgical instruments will then be superimposed on the 3D map provided by the CAS. These applications have their greatest application in the surgery of malignant brain disease, where the target lesion may be deeply seated and not visible to the operating surgeon (See Figure 4.3 Chapter 4).

Laparoscopic and robotic minimally invasive surgery

By limiting body trauma, minimally invasive techniques reduce the need for postoperative analgesia, accelerate convalescence and lead to lower complication rates when compared to open surgery. Endoscopic techniques are now routinely employed in colorectal cancer, gynaecology and the removal of some peripheral lung cancers. Endoscopic mastectomy is a minimally invasive approach that may particularly benefit women with small breasts, in whom breast conserving surgery (BCS) may result in obvious breast asymmetry, inadequate resection margins and poor cosmesis (although rates of positive margins are higher than seen with skin-sparing or subcutaneous mastectomy).

Transanal endoscopic microsurgery (TEM) is an innovative technique that involves the use of a rectoscope inserted transanally, facilitating dissection under magnified views to enable precise excision. TEM local surgical excision has been shown to lead to better functional outcomes when compared to major transabdominal colorectal resection. It may be a good option for frail patients with early disease, in whom major abdominal surgery carries significant risks.

On the basis of current evidence, the National Institute for Health and Clinical Excellence (NICE) has endorsed the use of laparoscopy as an alternative to open surgery in patients with colorectal cancer.

Laparoscopy is complicated by a two-dimensional view, leading to a loss of depth perception for the surgeon, who necessarily operates in three-dimensional space. The fulcrum effect (counterintuitive internal motion of the working tip relative to the instrument handle) and the amplification of physiological tremor compound this problem. Robotic surgical systems such as the da Vinci system (see Figure 3.2) provide the surgeon with high-definition three-dimensional vision and motion scaling, such that normal motions at the working console are translated to smaller movements at the working tip. Physiological tremor filtration and a seated position help to reduce fatigue in the operating surgeon. This may have particular advantages in situations where access is limited and the potential for nerve damage is high (e.g. radical prostatectomy).

Margins

A fundamental oncological principle is the aim of removing the entire tumour with a clear margin. The pathological evaluation of the surgical resection margin is of great importance. This 'surgical classification' requires the pathologist to prepare the operative specimen slides such that the distance from the tumour tissue to the circumferential resection margin of the specimen may be assessed. Resections may be classified according to their margins

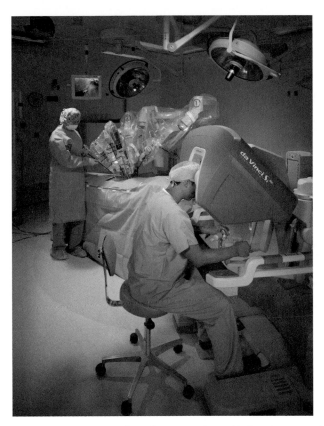

Figure 3.2 Robotic surgery allows the surgeon (seated in figure) to remotely control the fine movements of the multiple arms of the operating robot (rear of picture). Picture courtesy of Intuitive Health.

Table 3.3 Definitions of oncological resection according to margin.

Resection	Definition
R0	Complete removal of all tumour, with microscopic examination of margins showing no malignant cells
R1	Postoperative histopathology demonstrates that the margins of the resected lesion show tumour cells when viewed microscopically
R2	Macroscopic tumour is known to have been left behind at the time of surgery

(see Table 3.3). Definitions of adequate margin vary between disease sites and, with the exception of malignant melanoma, there have been very few randomised trials of margin size.

Even in the common case of breast cancer there is controversy as to how large the margin should be. In screen-detected breast cancer, the surgeon may not be able to 'see' the cancerous lesion as distinct from surrounding normal breast tissues. In that case, the specimen is localised by wires placed by radiologists and then x-rayed in the operating theatre. On reviewing the x-ray, the surgeon may decide on further excision of the breast cavity walls.

Function and reconstruction

The bigger the margin the surgeon takes, the more healthy tissue is necessarily removed. This leads to problems in both cosmesis and function. Modern surgery aims to combine oncological principles with plastic surgical methods to give the best functional and cosmetic outcomes (oncoplastic surgery).

In breast cancer, oncoplastic procedures enable greater volumes of tissue to be excised without deformity by reshaping the breast contour. In cases requiring mastectomy, there are multiple techniques to reconstruct the breast either at the time of cancer surgery (immediate breast reconstruction, IMBR) or as a delayed procedure.

Breast reconstruction is known to improve psychological morbidity and quality of life, and should be offered to all patients requiring mastectomy. IMBR combines procedures and thus avoids a second general anaesthetic. It allows potential preservation of the native skin envelope, giving improved cosmesis. However, it also leaves the patient with less decision-making time regarding their ideal reconstruction, and worse still, adjuvant therapy may be delayed by surgical complications (e.g. seroma, infection, etc.). Delayed reconstruction avoids this latter risk and gives the patient more time with her surgeon to determine the optimal reconstructive approach.

Reconstruction may be with an expander (using a part-saline/part-silicone implant) or autologous (using the patient's own tissue), or a hybrid of the two.

Implants are placed beneath the pectoralis muscle. Expandable implants have a port tunnelled to a subcutaneous location that can be accessed in order to progressively expand them in outpatients. Implants can be complicated by the development of fibrous capsule around them, which can contract ('capsular contracture'), leading to pain and implant distortion in severe cases. These reconstructions can be revised by capsulotomy (incisions in the fibrous capsule) or capsulectomy. Cosmesis may be improved by inserting a more natural, tear-drop, fixed-volume silicone implant.

Autologous reconstruction techniques isolate a paddle of skin, muscle and fascia (myocutaneous flap) or skin and subcutaneous tissue without muscle (myosubcutaneous flap). These flaps can be raised on their host blood supply, leaving the vessels intact ('pedicled flap'), or else the vasculature to the flap can be disconnected and anastomosed to local vessels using microsurgical techniques ('free flap').

In breast surgery, the latissimus dorsi (LD) pedicled flap is commonly used as it avoids the need for microsurgical techniques. The LD muscle is raised on a paddle of overlying skin and dissected from the muscle, while thoracodorsal blood supply is preserved. LD reconstruction can be used in isolation (autologous LD) or in combination with an implant. The donor scar is hidden in the bra line and patients do not typically notice any functional limitation from the procedure. Complications include donor-site seroma formation (40% of patients).

Free flaps are usually based on abdominal tissues such as the deep inferior epigastric perforator flap (DIEP). This flap leads to less weakness and hernia formation than older procedures such as the transverse abdominis muscle flap (TRAM).

In other areas, free flap surgery may be used to restore function as well as cosmesis. In head and neck cancer surgery, the radial forearm free flap (RFFF) is commonly used to repair functional deficit and to close the gap left after major resection. This flap can

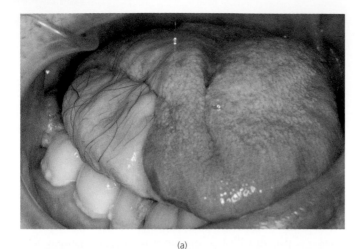

(a)

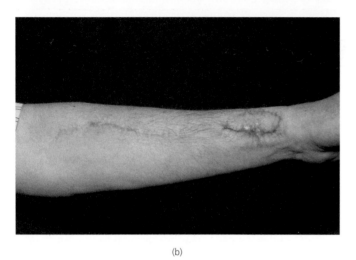

(b)

Figure 3.3 The use of tissue flaps allows the removal of tissue with replacement and restoration of function. In this case, (a) the right side of the tongue has been removed and replaced with a paddle of skin and muscle from the forearm (b). This gives the patient near-normal speech and swallowing.

restore speech and swallow functions after oral cancer excision (see Figure 3.3). If mandible is also resected, a composite flap using bone and muscle (e.g. fibula) may be harvested and used. Reconstruction may involve reconnecting the upper oesophagus using a free flap from the thigh, which is fashioned into a tube to replace the resected tissue.

Bowel and bladder surgery may cause loss of function. Following resection of diseased bowel, an anastomosis (formation of a join between two healthy ends of bowel) is fashioned using either a stapling device or sutures. The specific operative strategy depends on whether a sphincter-preserving operation is technically feasible and appropriate. If sphincter preservation is not possible, an abdominoperineal resection of the rectum (APR) is conducted, in which the rectum is excised along with the anus and a permanent stoma is formed. The perineal defect may need closure with a tissue flap (e.g. inferior gluteal artery perforator or 'iGAP' flap). In this setting, a stoma is an unavoidable consequence of cancer surgery.

If sphincter preservation is deemed appropriate then an anterior resection of the rectum is conducted with a total mesorectal excision (TME). Here the use of a specially designed circular stapling device facilitates anastomosis of descending colon and the lower rectum.

After urological surgery, such as cystectomy or cystourethrectomy, a urinary diversion into a stoma is necessary.

Emergency surgery

Most cancer surgery is planned electively, but some – colorectal cancer in particular – may present initially to the surgeon as an emergency with obstruction or perforation. Preoperative principles also apply to the patient requiring emergency surgery. Bowel preparation is contraindicated in the presence of intestinal obstruction and the emergency surgeon may instead choose to use an on-table technique if they are planning to perform a primary anastomosis. A temporary stoma is often fashioned under these circumstances, and in some cases the rectal stump is oversewn (Hartmann's procedure). Despite the feasibility of GI reconstruction, up to 50% of frail and elderly patients are deemed unfit for reversal of Hartmann's and so a stoma created with temporary intent sadly becomes permanent by default.

Further reading

Ellis, H., Calne, R. & Watson, C. (2011) *Lecture Notes: General Surgery*, 12th edn. Wiley-Blackwell, Chicester.

Glechner, A., Wöckel, A., Gartlehner, G., Thaler, K., Strobelberger, M., Griebler, U. & Kreienberg, R. (2012) Sentinel lymph node dissection only versus complete axillary lymph node dissection in early invasive breast cancer: a systematic review and meta-analysis. *European Journal of Cancer*. doi:10.1016/j.ejca.2012.09.01.

National Health Service (2012) Enhanced recovery: a better journey for patients and a better deal for the NHS, http://www.improvement.nhs.uk /enhancedrecovery/ (last accessed 8 March 2013).

National Institute of Health and Clinical Excellence (2006) Technology appraisal TA105: colorectal cancer – laparoscopic surgery (review), http://guidance.nice.org.uk/TA105 (last accessed 8 March 2013).

CHAPTER 4

Surgery for Metastatic Disease

Timothy W.R. Briggs[1], Elizabeth J. Gillott[1], Lewis W. Thorne[2], and Long R. Jiao[3]

[1]Royal National Orthopaedic Hospital, Stanmore, UK
[2]The National Hospital for Neurology and Neurosurgery, London, UK
[3]Imperial College London, London, UK

OVERVIEW

- Surgery is used increasingly in the palliation of patients
- Surgery of metastatic disease may achieve a cure in some settings, such as colorectal cancer
- Staging of the disease is an important tool for predicting prognosis and determining treatment
- Performance scores can be useful in guiding treatment decisions
- Ablative therapy may be used for those patients for whom surgery is not an option
- Fixation of impending fractures yields better results than fixation of pathological fractures of long bones

Introduction

Although previously the mainstay of radical treatment for primary cancer, surgery is increasingly used in the treatment of patients with secondary/metastatic disease for both palliation and in some cases attempted cure.

Sites of metastasis can vary between cancers, although some sites are more common, such as bone, liver and lung (Table 4.1). Cancer spreads via local invasion (nearby normal tissue is replaced by cancer cells) or by distant spread via blood or the lymphatic system.

Micrometastases are 'small numbers of cancer cells that have spread from the primary tumour to other parts of the body and are too few to be picked up in a screening or diagnostic test' (National Cancer Institute). They are often defined as having a size <2 mm. Macrometastases are defined as 'clinically detectable nodal metastases confirmed by therapeutic lymphadenectomy or when nodal metastasis exhibits gross extracapsular extension' (Balch *et al.* 2000).

Oligometastatic disease

Very limited secondary disease, on a spectrum between purely localised and widely metastatic, may be termed 'oligometastatic'. This is clinically significant, as patients with oligometastatic disease are potentially amenable to a curative therapeutic strategy.

Table 4.1 The 10 most common cancers in the UK (2007/08 figures), with the most common sites of metastases.

Cancer	% all cancers (UK)	Incidence	UK deaths/year	Common sites of metastasis
Bladder	4%	10 300	5000	Brain, lung
Breast	16%	47 000	12 116	Bone, brain, liver, lung
Colorectal	13%	39 991	16 260	Liver, lung
Kidney	3%	8757	3848	Bone, brain, lung
Lung	13%	40 800	35 260	Bone, brain, liver
Melanoma	4%	11 770	2070	Brain, liver
Non-Hodgkin lymphoma	4%	11 861	4438	N/A
Oesophageal	3%	7966	7606	Liver
Pancreatic	3%	8085	7781	Liver
Prostate	12%	37 051	10 170	Bone, brain, lung

Surgery for patients with metastases

The decision regarding surgery and treatment intent should be made by the multidisciplinary team (MDT), taking into account the known natural history of the disease, other available treatment options and the patient's performance status (see Box 4.1). Realistic expectations and potential risks must be discussed.

Box 4.1 **Preoperative considerations**

- Diagnosis.
- Patient evaluation/performance status/comorbidities.
- Stage of disease/life expectancy.
- Time since diagnosis of primary disease.
- Location of primary and secondary lesion.
- What treatment has already been given:
  - resection of the primary;
  - chemotherapy;
  - radiotherapy.
- Whether lesion represents a solitary or one of multiple metastatic lesions.
- Risk/benefit of the surgery and associated anaesthetic.
- Magnitude of proposed surgery and the patient's ability to rehabilitate from it.
- Intent of surgery.
- Patient's wishes.

ABC of Cancer Care, First Edition.
Edited by Carlo Palmieri, Esther Bird and Richard Simcock.
© 2013 John Wiley & Sons, Ltd. Published 2013 by John Wiley & Sons, Ltd.

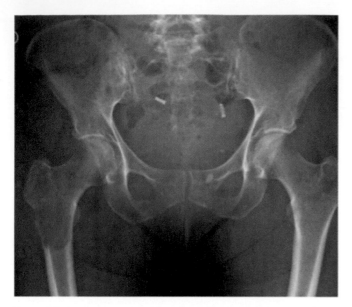

Figure 4.1 Anterior–posterior plain radiograph showing right proximal femur with a subtrochanteric pathological fracture due to metastases.

Table 4.2 Mirels scoring-based treatment recommendations (1989). Bone lesions are given a score (a) on the basis of their characteristics. This is then used to help determine treatment strategy (b).

(a) Scoring system

Score	1	2	3
Pain	Mild	Moderate	Mechanical pain
Lesion size/diameter of bone involved	<1/3	1/3–2/3	>2/3
Lesion type (blastic vs lytic)	Blastic	Mixed	Lytic
Anatomic site	Upper limb	Lower limb	Peritrochanteric (proximal femur)

(b) Treatment strategy

Total Mirels score	Risk of fracture	Recommended treatment
≥9	Impending	Prophylactic fixation
8	Borderline	Consideration of fixation
≤7	Not impending	Nonoperative management

Metastases to bone

Metastatic bone disease can have a major impact on quality of life, causing pain, fractures (acute and impending) (Figure 4.1) and loss of function. Surgery is indicated in cases of fracture or impending fracture or of intractable pain. In these circumstances, surgery will give local tumour control and restore function and mechanical stability.

Not all bony metastases require surgical treatment, and some may be adequately treated with radiotherapy (see Chapter 7).

Renal cell carcinoma

Solitary bone metastases from renal cell carcinoma (RCC) can be considered for radical resection given the long natural history of the disease; this involves removal of the mass, including bone, often using endoprostheses.

These lesions are often hypervascular, and therefore preoperative embolisation is recommended to counter the potential for life-threatening haemorrhage during surgery.

Orthopaedic fixation for bone disease

A clear indication for operative intervention is pathological fracture of a weight-bearing long bone; however, prophylactic fixation of impending fractures yields better outcomes. Identifying which lesions may go on to fracture can be difficult. The Mirels scoring system can be used to predict risk of pathological fracture associated with metastases in long bones. Scores are based on the x-ray appearance, which then helps to direct treatment (Table 4.2).

Operative management may be more complicated than general traumatic fracture fixation. Consideration needs to be given to the possibility of other metastases and the fact that soft tissue may be involved by tumour. The tumour may be close to or involve the

neurovascular bundle of the limb. Bone healing of pathological fractures is generally impaired. Surgery allows for tissue samples to be sent for pathological examination.

A total bone scintigraphic evaluation using technetium-99m (bone scan) may be undertaken in order to detect additional metastases that also require surgical treatment (Figure 4.2).

Fixation of long bones

Orthopaedic fixation usually utilises an intramedullary nail, as this involves relatively small wounds and minimal bone destruction. Since it leaves the soft tissue envelope *in situ*, it offers protection against displacement of the fracture. The fixation method chosen must be planned to be robust enough to outlive the patient and allow mobilisation.

Orthopaedic implants offer structural stability. While cement can be added if required, bone graft is not often used, as it relies upon bone healing to function. In the presence of sizeable bone destruction, resection and endoprostheses may be required. Excision of the lesion tissue also permits subsequent pathological examination.

Spinal metastases

The spine is the usual site of bony metastases, the thoracic area being the most common.

Patients with spinal metastases are at risk of developing metastatic spinal cord compression (MSCC). This is an oncological emergency (see Chapter 12) and patients should be informed of the action that must be taken if they develop symptoms.

Plain films should not be used to make or exclude the diagnosis of MSCC. Whole-spine magnetic resonance imaging (MRI) should be performed in order to determine whether spinal metastases are present and to what degree the cord or cauda equina is compressed. A computed tomography (CT) scan can be used to assess for stability.

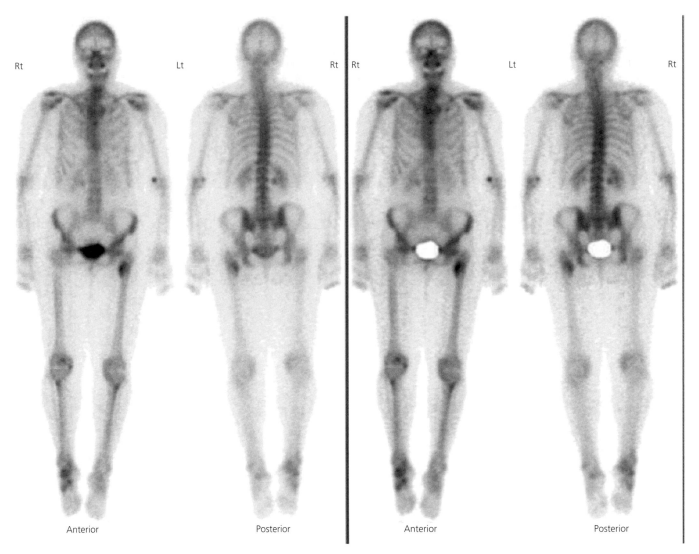

Rt   Lt   Rt   Rt   Lt   Rt

Anterior   Posterior   Anterior   Posterior

Figure 4.2 Nuclear magnetic bone scintigraphy showing an 8 cm metastatic lesion, left proximal femoral metadiaphyseal region originating at the level of the lesser trochanter. Scan shows aggressive bone destruction resulting in mild endosteal scalloping and expansion of the lateral cortex, but no cortical destruction. (The injection site can be seen in the left antecubital fossa. Degenerative changes are present in the right knee, right ankle and midfoot region, and also in the acriomoclavicular joints.)

Myelography can be used if MRI and CT are contraindicated, but technical expertise must be available to perform urgent decompression, as patients with MSCC may deteriorate following myelography.

A meta-analysis comparing surgery versus conventional radiotherapy on the ambulatory status of patients with MSCC found that patients receiving surgery were 30% more likely to be ambulatory after treatment as compared to those receiving radiotherapy alone. Surgery should therefore always be considered.

Treatment options

All patients with MSCC should be offered dexamethasone (loading dose of at least 16 mg) as soon as possible, providing it is not contraindicated. They should continue to receive a short course of 16 mg dexamethasone daily while treatment is being planned. Doses should be reduced gradually over 5–7 days. Blood glucose levels should be monitored while patients are receiving corticosteroids. Dexamethasone is contraindicated in patients with a significant suspicion of lymphoma.

A Cochrane review suggested that for selected ambulant patients with stable spines, radiotherapy alone may suffice. As with long-bone fractures, prophylactic fixation can be considered if the spine is viewed as unstable. Nonambulant patients may benefit from decompressive surgery before radiotherapy.

Spinal surgery

Surgery is indicated for mechanical sequelae of spinal metastases in carefully selected patients (see Box 4.2). There are a variety of fixation methods available, depending on the realistic goals; these are generally decompression of the spinal cord and nerves, stabilisation of the spine, correction of deformity where possible and prevention of local recurrence.

Box 4.2 **Indications for surgical treatment of spinal metastases**

Spinal instability:

- >50% vertebral body collapse;
- two or more adjacent levels involved.

Progressive impingement on the spinal canal and compression of the spinal cord by:

- radioresistant tumour (sarcoma, lung, renal cell, colorectal);
- recurrent tumour having already been treated with maximum irradiation;
- bone or soft-tissue debris extruding into canal as a result of progressive deformity.

Progressive kyphotic deformity:

- intact posterior structures but intractable pain due to mechanical causes;
- disruption of posterior elements and progressive shear deformity.

Vertebroplasty and kyphoplasty

Some patients may be deemed suitable for minimally invasive techniques, which are often helpful in providing pain relief. At vertebroplasty, surgical cement is injected percutaneously into the vertebral body. With kyphoplasty, a balloon is first introduced into the vertebral body and then inflated, creating a space. The balloon is then removed and the cement is introduced into the new space. These procedures should be performed in a facility where there is good access to spinal surgery.

Brain metastases

The aim of management is to ameliorate symptoms and, where possible, to prevent death by progression of cerebral disease. Again, the key determinants are: performance status, age and status of underlying disease. In well selected patients, survival can be measured in years.

Without treatment, most patients with brain metastases will die within a month. High-dose steroids reduce mass effect from associated cerebral oedema and will increase median survival by around 2 months. For patients with advanced systemic disease, this can provide sufficient palliation for the remainder of their lives, without the toxicity and hazard of other interventions. Whole-brain radiotherapy (WBRT) provides good local control and usually extends life to 3–4 months. This remains a good option for patients who are of a reasonably good performance status but have a poor overall prognosis from their primary disease, or for patients with multiple metastases.

Patients expected to survive more than 6 months, usually with controlled primary disease, good performance status, younger age and a limited number of metastases, may be suitable for surgical resection or stereotactic radiosurgery (SRS). Data would suggest that surgery and SRS are equivalent and can be used in combination. Surgical resection is the preferred management for solitary or large metastases. Functional MRI, fibre tracking, image guidance and

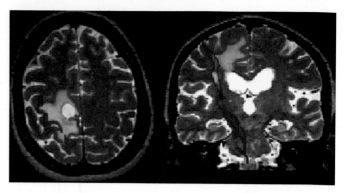

Figure 4.3 Functional MRI and DTI (Diffuser Tension Imaging) showing relationship of a cerebral metastasis to the motor cortex and associated white matter tract demonstrating a potential safe surgical corridor. These images can be linked to intra-operative navigation systems showing the surgeon where in the brain they are relative to the patients scans.

awake surgery can be used in combination for surgical planning, but resection may be limited by tumour location (Figure 4.3).

SRS works by using converging beams of low-energy radiation to produce a 'hot spot' on the tumour, like focusing the sun's rays with a magnifying glass. This minimises the dose to surrounding tissue. Various machines are capable of delivering SRS. The Gamma Knife uses a hemispherical arrangement of collimators to focus radiation. A linear accelerator can be moved in fractions through a progressive arc to the same effect. The Cybernife uses a linear accelerator mounted on a robotic arm to allow multiple fractions to be delivered in one session. There are no data comparing the different modes of delivery, and all would seem to be equally effective. They are usually limited to lesions less than 2.5 cm in diameter.

WBRT can be used after SRS or surgery. Evidence suggests this leads to better local control, but there are concerns regarding early and late toxicity, particularly as they relate to cognition for longer survivors. The same studies show no difference in maintenance of independence and overall survival. For this reason, some centres choose to delay WBRT after surgery or SRS as a salvage procedure. Studies are ongoing to see if SRS after surgical resection is a better option in selected patients.

Liver metastases

Patients with liver (hepatic) metastases should be discussed at a specialist liver multidisciplinary meeting. Patients with solitary, multiple and bilobar disease, and who have had radical treatment of their primary cancer in the case of colorectal cancer, are considered to be candidates for liver resection.

The aim of liver resection is to remove all macroscopic disease, leaving clear margins and sufficient functioning liver. In order to determine whether this has been achieved, the surgeon will take into consideration the functional anatomy of the liver, using the Couinaud classification for example (Box 4.3).

If surgery is contraindicated (e.g. in the presence of widespread disease in nodes, lung or peritoneum or in the central nervous system (CNS)) or technically not possible, patients can be considered for ablative therapy. Ablation therapies attack the tumour lesion(s)

Box 4.3 **Couinaud classification of functional liver anatomy and relationship to resection**

- Divides the liver into eight independent segments.
- Each segment has its own:
  - vascular inflow;
  - vascular outflow;
  - biliary drainage.
- Independent segments can be resected without damaging those remaining.
- Viability is preserved by resecting along the lines of the vessels that define the peripheries of segments.
- Generally, resection lines parallel the hepatic veins on the periphery.
- The vascular inflow and biliary drainage through the centre of the segment are generally preserved.

Table 4.3 Ablation techniques.

Name	Ablation technique	Application
Cryotherapy	Liquid nitrogen or argon to freeze the cancerous cells. Probe placed directly into the tumour	Hepatic metastases
Laser interstitial thermal therapy (LITT)	Minimally invasive. Tissue death is induced by the heat generated from laser energy optical radiation. Magnetic resonance imaging (MRI) or computed tomography (CT) are used to accurately target the application	
Percutaneous ethanol injection (PEI)	Minimally invasive technique. Ethanol injected through the skin directly into liver tumour	Tumours <5 cm. Relatively ineffective in the treatment of liver (hepatic) metastases. Effective for single small hepatocellular carcinomas
Photodynamic therapy (PDT)	Injection of a photosensitising agent a few days before the laser is used to activate the agent, destroying the cells	
Radiofrequency ablation (RFA)	Insertion of a probe directly into the tumour and passing of high-frequency alternating current through it. The heat generated from the current causes tumour necrosis	Limited success in tumours >3 cm diameter

using a number of methods (see Table 4.3). An alternative technique is radioembolisation or selective internal radiotherapy (SIRT). This is a form of brachytherapy (chapter 7) and enables treatment of multiple sites of disease within the liver. The procedure involves injecting microspheres containing the pure β-emitter, yttrium-90 (SIR-Spheres), via a transfemoral route into the arterial supply of the liver. Given hepatic metastases derive their blood flow from the arterial vasculature the microspheres become lodged in the malignant microvasculature, so delivering high doses of ionising radiation to the tumour whilst minimizing radiation exposure to the normal liver. SIRT is used in the treatment of hepatocellular carcinoma as well as colorectal liver metastasis.

Lung metastases

Approximately 50% of all patients with metastatic cancer will develop a malignant pleural effusion. Fluid is first drained either thoracoscopically (under general anaesthetic (GA) or sedation) or by inserting a chest drain (thoracostomy) under local anaesthetic. In order to prevent reaccumulation, a pleurodesis can be performed by introducing a sclerosant into the cavity.

Some patients may benefit from surgical resection of lung metastases (pulmonary metastasectomy), including those with solid tumours. Metastasectomy can be achieved using minimally invasive video-assisted techniques, reducing the impact of major thoracic surgery. Pulmonary metastasectomy cases are reported to the International Registry of Lung Metastases, set up in 1991. Despite the frequency of pulmonary metastasectomy, there are currently no randomised trials evaluating its benefit.

Further reading

Balch, C.M., Buzaid, A.C., Atkins, M.B., Cascinelli, N., Coit, D.G., Fleming, I.D. *et al.* (2000) A new American Joint Committee on Cancer staging system for cutaneous melanoma. *Cancer*, **88(6)**, 1484–1491.

Dick, E.A., Taylor-Robinson, S.D., Thomas, H.C. & Gedroyc, W.M.W. (2002) Ablative therapy for liver tumours. *Gut*, **50**, 733–739.

Garden, O.J., Reese, M., Poston, G.J., Mirza, D., Saunders, M., Ledermann, J. *et al.* (2006) Guidelines for resection of colorectal cancer liver metastases. *Gut*, **55 (Suppl. 3)**, iii1–8.

Hart, M.G., Grant, R., Walker, M. & Dickinson, H.O. (2005) Surgical resection and whole brain radiation therapy versus whole brain radiation therapy alone for single brain metastases. *Cochrane Database of Systematic Reviews*. doi:10.1002/14651858.CD003292.pub2.

Shaw, P.H.S. & Agarwal, R. (2004) Pleurodesis for malignant pleural effusions. *Cochrane Database of Systematic Reviews*, **1**. doi:10.1002/14651858 .CD002916.pub2.

Tokuhashi, Y., Matsuzaki, H., Toriyama, S., Kawano, H. & Ohsaka, S. (1990) Scoring system for the preoperative evaluation of metastatic spine tumor prognosis. *Spine*, **15(11)**, 1110–1113.

CHAPTER 5

Chemotherapy

Catherine Harper-Wynne[1] *and Catherine M. Kelly*[2]

[1]Maidstone Hospital, Barming, Kent, UK
[2]Mater Misericordiae University Hospital, Dublin, Ireland

OVERVIEW

- Chemotherapy may be delivered as an curative, primary/neoadjuvant, adjuvant or palliative treatment
- Drugs are available as both oral and intravenous formulations and the development of central venous access devices allows safer administration as well as the potential for administration outside of a specialist cancer centre setting. In certain circumstance chemotherapy may also be given intrathecally or via intraperionteal route
- Cancer chemotherapy drugs may be classified according to their cellular mode of action and may be cell-cycle or non-cell-cycle specific

---

Introduction

Chemotherapy refers to a group of DNA-damaging agents, which by their cytotoxic action induce cell death or apoptosis. This contrasts with cytostatic agents, such as antiendocrine treatments, in which the predominant effect is on reducing cell proliferation (see Chapter 9). The term 'systemic anticancer therapy' (SACT) has been used to encompass all systemic treatments administered to patients as part of their cancer care. The first patient was treated with intravenous (IV) chemotherapy (nitrogen mustard) on 27 August 1942 (Box 5.1) and since then there has been an exponential growth in the use and development of chemotherapy, such that the treatment has its own branch of medical specialisation: medical oncology. A number of chemotherapy agents currently in use have been derived from natural sources such as plants and marine sponges (Figure 5.1).

Box 5.1 **First patient treated with intravenous chemotherapy**

After the entry of the USA into the Second World War, the United States Office of Scientific Research and Development sponsored research to explore antidotes to potential chemical warfare agents at Yale School of Medicine. Work by Gilman and Goodman with

---

ABC of Cancer Care, First Edition.
Edited by Carlo Palmieri, Esther Bird and Richard Simcock.
© 2013 John Wiley & Sons, Ltd. Published 2013 by John Wiley & Sons, Ltd.

nitrogen mustard led them to conclude that these agents might serve as a potential therapy of malignant lymphoid disease. Dr Gustaf E. Lindskog, Assistant Professor of Surgery at Yale, was approached by Gilman and Goodman with a view to performing a clinical study.

The first recipient of IV systemic chemotherapy was a 47-year-old male Polish immigrant to the USA named 'JD', who worked in a ball bearing factory. He had been diagnosed with a lymphosarcoma in 1941 and underwent a number of radiotherapy treatments. In August 1942 he was admitted to New Haven Hospital with axillary lymphadenopathy, dysphagia and weight loss. He was approached and agreed to receive intravenous chemotherapy – nitrogen mustard – which at the time was referred to as 'lymphocidin' and 'X' for reasons of secrecy. On 27th August 1942 he was commenced on his first of 10 daily injections. There was a significant improvement in his lymphadenopathy, and a biopsy of a right axillary node showed fibrous tissue and chronic inflammatory cells, but no tumour tissue. He subsequently underwent further chemotherapy treatments but died in December 1942. Post mortem revealed lymphosarcoma in cervical and axillary lymph nodes and aplasia of the bone marrow with replacement by fat.

The case of JD highlights some principles which still hold true today:

1 Multidisciplinary team meeting (MDTM) to discuss cases and management.
2 Patient altruism and involvement in clinic research.
3 Proof of concept that intravenous chemotherapy will result in tumour regression.
4 Development of chemoresistance to drugs after multiple doses.
5 Requirement for bloods prior to further treatments.
6 Benefit must be weighted up against side effects.

The secrecy surrounding the research meant that the results were not published until 1946 (Goodman *et al.* 1946).

Treatment settings

Chemotherapy may be given as the first cancer treatment for a patient and can substitute or precede surgery.

Curative Chemotherapy

Chemotherapy may be given with curative intent in some cancers such as testicular and ovarian germ cell tumours and lymphomas. In such cases the disease can be widespread and metastatic.

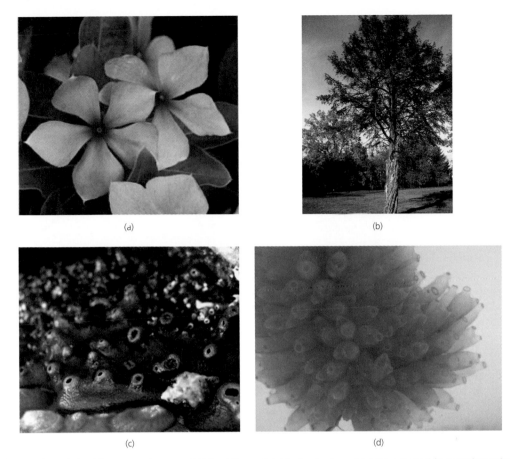

(a)

(b)

(c)

(d)

Figure 5.1 Chemotherapy drugs derived from natural sources. (a) Vincristine and vinblastine (a vinca alkloid) are derived from *Catharanthus roseus* (Madagascar periwinkle), formerly called *Vinca rosea*. (b) Paclitaxel (Taxol) was originally discovered in the bark of the Pacific yee tree, *Taxus brevifolia*. It was found that the endophytic fungi in the bark synthesised the drug. (c) Halichondrion B (Eribulin) was derived from the marine sponge, *Halichondria okada Kadota*. (d) Trabectedin (Yondelis) was derived from the sea squirt, *Ecteinascidia turbinata*.

Neoadjuvant/Primary chemotherapy

Neoadjuvant chemotherapy aims to reduce the size of the tumour or 'downstage' to improve surgical results and patient outcomes (e.g. in breast cancer to avoid mastectomy). Neoadjuvant therapy is commonly used in rectal cancer, where it is often combined with radiotherapy to improve tumour shrinkage. Occasionally, such as in the frail patient, where surgery is deemed inappropriate, chemotherapy may be used for palliation, but frequently a patient unfit for surgery will also not be suitable for chemotherapy. Neoadjuvant therapy is commonly used in rectal cancer, where it is often combined with radiotherapy to improve tumour shrinkage.

Occasionally, such as in the frail patient, where surgery is deemed inappropriate, chemotherapy may be used for palliation, but frequently a patient unfit for surgery will also not be suitable for chemotherapy.

Such treatments can also be used for a short period, for example 2 weeks, in the research setting and are known as 'window of opportunity' studies. These trials allow researchers to investigate changes in biomarkers (see Chapter 11).

Adjuvant chemotherapy

Chemotherapy is frequently delivered adjuvantly after surgery to eradicate both local and systemic microscopic disease. Survival benefits have been seen with this approach in many randomised controlled trials. Adjuvant chemotherapy is often given for 3–6 months following 4–6 weeks of surgical recovery. This strategy is common in breast, colon, gastrooesophageal, ovarian and lung cancers.

Palliative chemotherapy

Palliative chemotherapy is used for incurable advanced cancers, but where trials have shown benefit with regard to overall survival or improvement in quality of life and symptom control. Palliative chemotherapy is offered to patients who have a good general health and whom the clinician judges will be able to tolerate the toxicity of treatment. A general principle is that a patient should have an expected prognosis of at least 3 months in order for treatment to be considered. In several tumour types, patients may have several sequential 'lines' (treatment courses) of chemotherapy, some of which may be in the research setting.

NHS cancer strategies and chemotherapy

Since the advent of the NHS Cancer Plan in 2000, there has been a drive to improve cancer outcomes across all tumour types. There have been multiple strands to this approach, including improvement in chemotherapy access, delivery and toxicity management. A choice agenda has been introduced to influence where chemotherapy can be given, including ambulatory and home health care, and also to drive improvements in information for patients and carers. The formation of Cancer Networks and the use of National Peer Review sought to protocolise chemotherapy regimens for all tumour types and try to ensure that there were not large variations of practice.

Management of chemotherapy toxicity has been scrutinised following the National Confidential Enquiry into Patient Outcome and Death (NCEPOD) report on 30-day mortality following SACT. There has been criticism related to the management of acute toxicity of chemotherapy. Following this report, the National Cancer Action Team (NCAT) has recommended the development of Acute Oncology Teams with expertise to manage the complications and toxicity of chemotherapy.

Patient information has also been addressed, and Macmillan Cancer Support and Cancer Research UK are developing a personalised patient prescription strategy to give further information to patients regarding their cancer treatments.

Administration of chemotherapy

SACT involves a wide range of agents, some of which can be given orally, such as the prodrug Capecitabine and some newer small-molecule agents (see Chapter 10), the intrathecal and intraperitoneal route can also be used. However, the vast majority of chemotherapy is administered intravenously.

Oral administration

Oral chemotherapy is often preferred by patients for the sake of convenience, although the oral formulation is not always less toxic. Where similar efficacy allows a choice between intravenous (IV) and oral, careful evaluation is required. Alongside convenience, other factors such as compliance and the psychological impact of self-administration at home, often for several days or weeks, must be assessed.

IV administration

This can involve several methods, depending on the frequency and duration of the regimen and an evaluation of the patient's peripheral vein quality. IV delivery is inconvenient but the vesicant (blistering) nature of many chemotherapy agents requires secure and careful IV access.

IV access

Many regimens are of a relatively short duration (a few months) and involve bolus or short infusional delivery (up to a few hours). In these situations, if there is good vein quality and no contraindications, single-use access using a standard peripheral cannula is appropriate. There are situations, however, in which single-use access is not suitable and a central venous access device (CVAD) is preferable (Figure 5.2). These devices are long-term indwelling and thus afford reliable IV access, preventing failure of chemotherapy delivery and thus delay of treatment. The three main CVADs

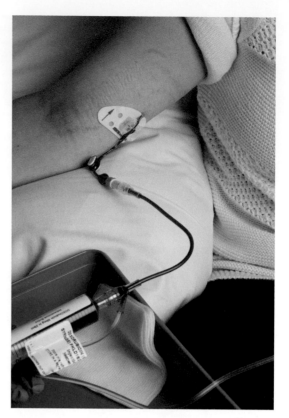

Figure 5.2 Vesicant drugs and CVADs. Chemotherapy drugs can be highly toxic to veins and tissues. Here a nurse wearing protective gloves is administering doxorubicin (an anthracycline) using a peripherally inserted central catheter (PICC) line sited in the patient's arm; the distal end of the PICC line will deliver the chemotherapy directly into the large superior vena cava.

are summarised in Table 5.1. The main complications are infection/sepsis rate, thrombosis and pneumothorax.

Particular attention should be given to certain skin and venous complications relating to the use of IV administration of chemotherapy. Patient education is key to early recognition and presentation of these conditions to improve outcome, together with early referral into the specialist centre.

Cellulitis can occur following local infection around the single-use cannula or CVAD insertion site. Bruising is not uncommon with single-use peripheral cannula insertion through repeated attempts.

Discomfort and pain can develop along the vein, with associated skin changes, as a result of irritation by a chemotherapy agent. Certain agents are more damaging than others. Management of these vesicant drugs involves pain and inflammation control using nonsteroidal anti-inflammatory drugs (NSAIDs), as well as the use of antibiotics if infection is suspected.

Extravasation is a leakage of chemotherapy into the subcutaneous tissues rather than intravenously, usually due to cannulation failure. Some powerful vesicants (e.g. the anthracyclines and the vinca alkaloids) will cause pain, erythema, inflammation and discomfort, which, if left undiagnosed or inappropriately treated, can lead to necrosis and functional loss of the tissue and limb concerned. Extravasation risk is reduced by the use of a CVAD. Extravasation should be treated as a medical emergency. There are clear extravasation guidelines and kits in all clinical areas delivering SACT.

Table 5.1 Comparison of differing CVAD devices for chemotherapy.

	Peripherally inserted central catheter (PICC)	External catheters, e.g. Groshong and Hickman lines	Subcutaneous implanted venous access devices/ports
Device details	Inserted into a large peripheral vein either via the antecubital fossa or through ultrasound-guided placement into the basilic or cephalic vein in the upper arm Tip is located in the lower third of the superior vena cava	Require skin tunneling along the chest wall before coming to reside in the central vein Have externally placed lumens over the chest wall for access	Subcutaneously implanted venous access devices or ports are inserted either peripherally into a vein near the antecubital fossa or centrally directly into the subclavian or jugular vein Access diaphragm is located just under the skin
Why used	Continuous infusion of chemotherapy, i.e. >6-hour regimen Requires two lumens for delivery of simultaneous incompatible agents Needle phobia to repeated single-use cannula insertion	As per PICC Peripheral access not possible	As per external catheter
Advantages over other CVADs	Neglible risk of pneumothorax Relatively quick and easy to insert and can be inserted by trained nursing staff	Less risk of extravasation than with PICCs	No external cannulas to break Improved body image for certain groups of patients, e.g. adolescents Less restriction of movement than external catheters Can swim and bathe with minimal restriction Thrombotic and infection risk believed to be less than with external catheters Can remain in for longer than external catheter lines or PICCs, e.g. years Easier maintenance than external catheters
Complications/ disadvantages compared to other CVADs	More restrictive regarding arm movement compared to other CVADs Thrombotic and infection risk probably higher than for ports	Increased risk of pneumothorax compared to PICCs Thrombotic and infection risk higher than for ports Requires more skin tunneling than do ports	Increased risk of pneumothorax compared to PICCs Require access with a needle via the skin and are therefore problematic for needle-phobic patients Extravasation more of a hazard than with external catheters Most expensive to insert CVADs, requiring additional training that is not always available Usually require operation to insert

Intrathecal (IT) Administration

Chemotherapy can also be administered directly into the cerebrospinal fluid. This can be done via a lumbar puncture or an Ommaya reservoir (intraventricular catheter system). Only methotrexate, cytarabine and hydrocortisone can be given by the IT route. Such treatment is given as prophylaxis in tumours at high risk of involving the CNS (e.g. lymphoma) or as treatment for leptomeningeal metastases (e.g. breast cancer). In the UK strict rules govern the administration of chemotherapy agents via the IT route following deaths from the IT delivery of the highly neurotoxic vinca alkaloids.

Intraperitoneal Administration

Intraperitoneal chemotherapy is the administration of chemotherpy into the abdominal cavity via an indwelling catheter. It is used in the treatment of advanced stage ovarian cancer.

Modes of action of chemotherapy

Highly proliferative cancers are more sensitive to the effects of cytotoxic chemotherapy than those cancers with a low proliferative potential. Chemotherapy exerts its cytotoxic effect by targeting DNA or RNA directly (e.g. platinum compounds and other alkylating agents, anthracyclines), interfering or competing with the production of purines and pyrimidines (e.g. anthracyclines) or preventing the process of cell division via microtubule disruption (e.g. antimitotic agents) (Table 5.2). In contrast to targeted agents, chemotherapy can affect noncancerous proliferating cells, giving rise to common side effects (such as alopecia, gastrointestinal toxicity and bone marrow suppression) observed in patients receiving chemotherapy (see Chapter 6).

Chemotherapeutic agents can be classified as cell-cycle specific if they are most effective against proliferating cells (e.g. antimetabolites) or cell-cycle nonspecific if they have activity against both proliferating and nonproliferating cells (e.g. alkylating agents).

Dosing and schedule

Chemotherapy agents are typically dosed according to body surface area (calculated from height and weight). Doses should not be reduced in the obese patient as this might lead to underdosing. Carboplatin is dosed according to renal function, as it is renally excreted. All drugs may require planned dose reductions in the face of renal or hepatic impairment affecting metabolism of the drug. Some drugs have standard schedules for dose modification in the face of predictable toxicity (e.g. Capecitabine and plantar palmar erythema syndrome).

Table 5.2 Chemotherapeutic agents used to treat common cancer types.

Chemotherapy class (example of tumour types treated)	Mechanism of action	Common side effects
Antimetabolites		
5-fluorouracil (colon, rectal, hepatobiliary, breast)	*Antimetabolites are structurally similar to compounds that exist within the cell. They interfere with the synthesis of purines and pyrimidines or compete with them in RNA and DNA synthesis*	Gastrointestinal disturbance, nausea, vomiting, mucositis, bone marrow suppression, hand foot syndrome
Capecitabine (colon, rectal, hepatobiliary, breast)		Gastrointestinal disturbance, nausea, vomiting, hand foot syndrome
Gemcitabine (pancreatic, hepatobiliary, breast, ovarian, bladder)		Myelosuppression, nausea, vomiting, transient elevations in transaminases, proteinuria, haematuria
Fludarabine (chronic lymphocytic leukaemia, indolent non-Hodgkin lymphoma, hairy cell leukaemia)		Nausea, vomiting, gastrointestinal disturbance, myelosuppression
Cladribine (chronic lymphocytic leukaemia, non-Hodgkin lymphoma, hairy cell leukaemia)		Bone marrow suppression, fever
6-mercaptopurine (maintenance of remission in acute lymphoblastic leukaemia)		Bone marrow suppression, anorexia, nausea, vomiting and gastrointestinal disturbance, hepatotoxicity
Methotrexate (acute lymphocytic leukaemia, choriocarcinoma, Burkitt lymphoma, breast, head and neck)		Nausea, vomiting, gastrointestinal disturbance, stomatitis, myelosuppression
Antibiotics		
Bleomycin (testicular, squamous cell carcinomas, lymphomas)	*Antibiotics cause disruption of DNA through intercalation, inhibition of topoisomerases (I and II) and formation of free radicals*	'Bleomycin lung' pulmonary fibrosis, alopecia, mucocutaneous reactions, hypertrophic skin changes and hyperpigmentation
Doxorubicin (breast, lymphoma, lung, sarcoma, acute lymphocytic leukaemia)		Cardiac toxicity, nausea, vomiting, bone marrow suppression, stomatitis, gastrointestinal disturbance, alopecia
Epirubicin (breast, lymphoma, lung, sarcoma, acute lymphocytic leukaemia)		Cardiac toxicity, nausea, vomiting, bone marrow suppression, stomatitis, gastrointestinal disturbance, alopecia
Daunorubicin (breast, lymphoma, lung, sarcoma, acute lymphocytic leukaemia)		Cardiac toxicity, nausea, vomiting, bone marrow suppression, stomatitis, gastrointestinal disturbance, alopecia
Dactinomycin (Wilms tumour, gestastional choriocarcinoma, soft-tissue sarcoma)		Bone marrow suppression, nausea, vomiting, gastrointestinal disturbance, stomatitis, alopecia
Alkylating agents		
Cyclophosphamide	*These cytotoxic agents form covalent bonds with nucleophilic groups on various cellular constituents, including DNA*	Nausea, vomiting, gastrointestinal disturbance, bone marrow suppression, haemorrhagic cystitis, infertility, veno-occlusive disease, secondary malignancies
Ifosphamide		Nausea, vomiting, gastrointestinal disturbance, bone marrow suppression, haemorrhagic cystitis, infertility, veno-occlusive disease, secondary malignancies
Dacarbazine (melanoma)		Bone marrow suppression, nausea, vomiting
Melphalan (multiple myeloma)		Bone marrow suppression
Temozolamide (brain tumours, melanoma)		Bone marrow suppression, nausea, vomiting
Microtubule inhibitors		
Docetaxel (breast, prostate, lung)	*These agents disrupt the equilibrium between polymerised and depolymerised forms of the microtubules and thereby disrupt the ability of the mitotic spindle to partition DNA into the two daughter cells formed during cell division*	Nausea, vomiting, gastrointestinal disturbance, bone marrow suppression, peripheral neuropathy, fluid retention
Paclitaxel (breast, lung, ovarian)		Nausea, vomiting, gastrointestinal disturbance, bone marrow suppression, peripheral neuropathy, fluid retention
Vinblastine (testicular, lymphoma, lung)		Nausea, vomiting, gastrointestinal disturbance, phlebitis, cellulitis, myelopsuppressive
Vincristine (acute lymphoblastic leukaemia, Wilms tumour, Ewing soft-tissue sarcoma, Hodgkin and non-Hodgkin lymphomas)		Nausea, vomiting, gastrointestinal disturbance, phlebitis, cellulitis, peripheral neuropathy
Vinorelbine (breast, lung)		Bone marrow suppression
Platinums		
Cisplatin (germ cell tumours, head and neck, cervical, lung, upper gastrointestinal (GI) tumours)	*The mechanism of action of this class of chemotherapeutic agent is similar to that of alkylating agents. Intra- and interstrand crosslinks result in cytotoxic lesions that inhibit DNA replication and RNA synthesis*	Nausea, vomiting, gastrointestinal disturbance, nephrotoxicity, ototoxicity, neurotoxicity
Carboplatin (ovarian, lung, seminoma, breast)		Nausea, vomiting, gastrointestinal disturbance, nephrotoxicity, ototoxicity, neurotoxicity
Oxaliplatin (colorectal)		Nausea, vomiting, gastrointestinal disturbance, neurotoxicity

Chemotherapy schedules are built around the half lives of the drugs involved and crucially around the time taken for normal cells to recover (particularly their neutrophil count). Neutropenia is the cause of the most significant chemotherapy toxicities (see Chapters 6 and 12) and counts will usually reach a nadir 7–10 days after chemotherapy, before recovering by Day 21, leading to the commonly adopted 3-weekly schedules. In order to treat cancer more intensively, accelerated schedules have been developed in which neutrophil counts are maintained by granulocyte colony stimulating factors (GCSFs) and treatment may be delivered 2-weekly. Some chemotherapies show increased efficacy when given more frequently at lower doses (e.g. weekly paclitaxel or cisplatin).

The number of doses (cycles) delivered during a course of chemotherapy will vary according to the tumour being treated. Cycle number may be limited by the cumulative toxicity of the drug or by its efficacy. In the adjuvant setting it is common to deliver six cycles of treatment during a course. Cycle number may be low in very sensitive disease (e.g. a single cycle in adjuvant testicular treatments) or indefinite in well-tolerated palliative treatment (e.g. Capecitabine in metastatic breast cancer).

Combinations of chemotherapy are given, comprising agents from different classes and with different modes of action and toxicity. These combinations are designed to maximise cancer cell kill by using drugs with differing mechanisms, but they rely on the drugs having nonoverlapping toxicities such that the treatment is tolerable. Standardised treatment protocols specify the cytotoxic drug combination, dosing, treatment schedule and dose adjustments according to well-defined toxicity criteria. Supportive agents, such as antiemetics, antidiarrhoea medications and GCSF, are often incorporated into the protocol and given prophylactically (see Chapter 6).

Chemotherapy agents are now increasingly being used in combination with biological agents (see Chapter 10), where they may combine synergistically (e.g. taxanes given with Trastuzumab in HER-2 positive metastatic breast cancer).

Chemotherapy may be combined with radiotherapy, where it may act as a radiosensitiser (increasing the biological effectiveness of the treatment). Radiochemotherapy is now a very common radical treatment strategy, particularly in squamous cell cancers of the lung, head and neck, oesophagus, cervix and anus. The chemotherapy class used most commonly in combination with radiotherapy is the platinum agents (cisplatin and carboplatin).

Further reading

Department of Health (2000, 2002, 2005) *National Cancer Plans (2000, 2002, 2005)*, available from http://www.dh.gov.uk (last accessed 8 March 2013).

Goodman, L.G., Wintrobe, M.M., Dameshek, W., Goodman, M.J., Gilman, A. & McLennan, M.T. (1946) Nitrogen mustard therapy: use of methyl-bis(beta-chloroethyl)amine hydrochloride and tris(beta-chloroethyl)amine hydrochloride for Hodgkin's disease, lymphosarcoma, leukemia and certain allied and miscellaneous disorders. *Journal of the American Medical Association*, **132**, 126–132.

National Confidential Enquiry into Patient Outcome and Death (2008) For better, for worse? A review of the care of patients who died within 30 days of receiving systemic anti-cancer therapy, available from http://www.ncepod.org.uk (last accessed 8 March 2013).

Vardy, J., Engelhardt, K., Cox, K., Jacquet, J., McDade, A., Boyer, M. *et al.* (2004) Long-term outcome of radiological-guided insertion of implanted central venous access port devices (CVAPD) for the delivery of chemotherapy in cancer patients: institutional experience and review of the literature. *British Journal of Cancer*, **91(6)**, 1045–1049.

Wengström, Y., Margulies, A. & European Oncology Nursing Society Task Force (2008) European Oncology Nursing Society extravasation guidelines. *European Journal of Oncological Nursing*, **12(4)**, 357–361.

CHAPTER 6

Toxicities of Chemotherapy

Sacha Jon Howell[1], Alison Jones[2], and Colin R. James[3]

[1]University of Manchester, Institute of Cancer Studies; The Christie NHS Foundation Trust, Manchester, UK
[2]Royal Free Hospital and University College Hospital, London, UK
[3]Belfast Health and Social Care Trust; Northern Ireland Cancer Centre, Belfast City Hospital, Belfast, UK

> **OVERVIEW**
>
> - Chemotherapy causes a wide range of toxicities, affecting most organ systems. Rapidly proliferating cells are affected acutely
> - Acute gastrointestinal (GI) toxicities (diarrhoea and vomiting) can be successfully managed with appropriate supportive care
> - Effects on blood cells are predictable and manageable but can be fatal if overlooked or not managed promptly
> - There may be late effects on nerves, heart and lung tissue, as well as a risk of second malignancy

Introduction

The majority of acute toxicities seen with cytotoxic chemotherapy are secondary to its effects on rapidly dividing normal cells such as those in the bone marrow, skin and gastrointestinal (GI) tract. In addition, many cytotoxics can induce nausea and vomiting or neuropathies, due to direct effects on the central and peripheral nervous system, respectively. Most common acute toxicities are reversible following cessation of chemotherapy, although some acute toxicity, such as neuropathy, can result in permanent damage and ongoing symptoms and signs. Toxicities may be graded and scored according to agreed protocols, such as the Common Toxicity Criteria (CTC) produced by the European Organisation for Research and Treatment of Cancer (EORTC). Common toxicities are listed in Table 6.1.

Hair loss

Many chemotherapy drugs (particularly the anthracyclines and taxanes used commonly in the treatment of breast cancer) will cause total alopecia. The effect occurs due to interference with cell division at the hair root. Hair loss usually occurs within 2–4 weeks of the first dose of treatment, but regrowth will start as soon as chemotherapy is over if not before. The effect of the hair pushing through the scalp follicle will sometimes lead to a 'chemo curl'. While not physically harmful, alopecia can be a major source of

Table 6.1 Common and serious toxicities of chemotherapy and the drugs that cause them.

Toxicity	Principle cytotoxics associated with severe toxicity
Acute toxicity	
Nausea and vomiting	Platinum agents (esp. cisplatin), anthracyclines (doxorubicin, epirubicin), alkylating agents (e.g. cyclophosphamide, DTIC)
Anaemia (any cytotoxic can induce anaemia if given for prolonged periods)	Cisplatin, carboplatin, 5FU, topotecan, docetaxel, paclitaxel, etoposide, cyclophosphamide, doxorubicin, epirubicin
Thrombocytopenia (Many agents induce transient TCP – more common in combination regimens)	Platinum agents (esp. Carboplatin), gemcitabine, paclitaxel, 5FU/capecitabine
Neutropenia	Almost all cytotoxics, particularly in combination regimens. It is safer to assume that neutropenia can occur
Diarrhoea	Irinotecan, taxanes (esp. docetaxel), 5FU/capecitabine
Peripheral neuropathy (can be permanent)	Platinum agents (cisplatin > carboplatin), microtubule poisons including taxanes (docetaxel and paclitaxel), vinca alkaloids (e.g. vincristine and vinorelbine)
Chronic toxicity	
Pulmonary fibrosis	Bleomycin, busulphan and other alkylating agents, mitomycin C, taxanes (rarely)
Second cancers	Alkylating agents (e.g. cyclophosphamide), topoisomerase II inhibitors (e.g. etoposide) and anthracyclines (doxorubicin, epirubicin)
Cardiac failure	Anthracyclines (adriamycin, epirubicin)

emotional distress. Wigs should be supplied to patients who are expected to lose hair. Scalp hypothermia ('cold capping') uses a coolant fluid at $-5\,^{\circ}$C circulated via a special head gear immediately before, during and after chemotherapy to reduce blood flow to the scalp (see Figure 6.1). The cold cap is not always tolerated, nor is it 100% successful, but it may help some patients preserve hair. The charity My New Hair exists to support those upset by hair loss.

Through a similar effect on the keratin in the finger and toenails, many patients will experience growth arrest, leading to the appearance of horizontal Beau's lines in the nail or to fragile and brittle nails that lift and break (see Figure 6.2).

ABC of Cancer Care, First Edition.
Edited by Carlo Palmieri, Esther Bird and Richard Simcock.
© 2013 John Wiley & Sons, Ltd. Published 2013 by John Wiley & Sons, Ltd.

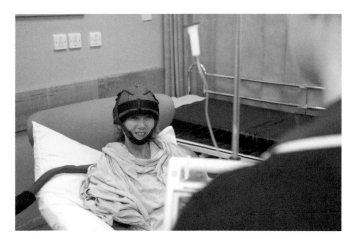

Figure 6.1 Scalp cooling device. The cooler pumps fluid through the device and circulates it through a tubing system incorporated in the patient's headgear.

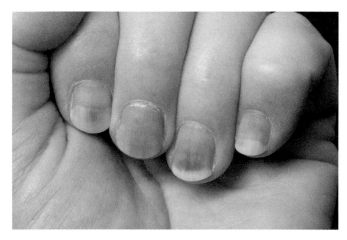

Figure 6.2 Nail changes on chemotherapy. In this patient, taxane chemotherapy has caused the nails to lift and become brittle. The chemotherapy stopped 6 weeks previously and there is now healthy growth at the nail bed.

Haematological toxicity

All three of the main cell lineages in the bone marrow can be affected by chemotherapy treatment. The commonest anaemia induced by cytotoxic agents is normochromic and normocytic, although a macrocytic anaemia can be induced by inhibitors of DNA synthesis such as 6MP, Ara-C and 5FU/capecitabine. Iron deficiency per se is not induced by chemotherapy but it is seen in many cancer patients due to chronic blood loss and/or poor nutritional status. In chemotherapy-induced anaemia, the haematinics (ferritin/B12/folate) are usually normal or raised, and treatment is most commonly blood transfusion if the patient is symptomatic or if chemotherapy is to continue. The toxic effects of chemotherapy drugs on the bone marrow are cumulative, and hence the incidence of anaemia increases with the duration of therapy. Erythropoietin can increase haemoglobin levels but has been associated with inferior outcomes in some trials and is therefore rarely used. Additional causes of chemotherapy-induced anaemia should also be

considered, including the nephrotoxicity induced by cisplatin and haemolytic anaemia induced by drugs such as mitomycin C.

Thrombocytopenia (TCP) is induced by many chemotherapy drugs. Patients should be made aware of this risk and counselled to look for signs of spontaneous bruising and bleeding and the development of a purpuric rash. Bleeding as a result of TCP often presents as persistent oozing from the mucous membranes of the gums or nose, rather than a heavy flow of blood. Treatment is with platelet transfusion if severe or in the presence of active bleeding. Concomitant anticoagulation may need to be discontinued during periods of severe TCP, but specialist haematological advice should be sought.

Myelosuppression is very common with cytotoxic chemotherapy. This results in a fall in circulating neutrophils (neutropenia) and tissue macrophages. As a result, patients with neutropenia are at significantly increased risk of bacterial infection. The longer the duration of neutropenia, the greater the risk of any infection, but also the greater the risk of atypical infections such as fungi, protozoa and unusual viruses. In general, prophylactic granulocyte colony stimulating factor (GCSF) is recommended for any patient receiving chemotherapy with a risk of febrile neutropenia of >20%, or of 10–20% and with additional risk factors such as comorbid conditions affecting infection risk, such as diabetes mellitus or chronic obstructive pulmonary disease (COPD). Patients should be warned of the potentially fatal outcome of febrile neutropenia and advised to check their temperature whenever they feel unwell after chemotherapy and, if it is elevated, to contact their treating centre urgently (see Chapter 12).

GI toxicity

The GI mucosa is highly proliferative and hence prone to chemotherapy-induced toxicity. The most common form is oral mucositis manifesting as pain, ulceration and swelling of the oral cavity. Mild symptoms, not limiting intake of food or drink, can be managed with mouthwashes to keep the mucosa clean; simple analgesia and barrier preparations can also help to reduce pain. More severe symptoms and signs of mucositis, particularly after high-dose chemotherapy, may necessitate admission for intravenous hydration and consideration of enteral or parenteral nutrition. In such cases, opiate analgesia is frequently required.

Diarrhoea is also a relatively common toxicity with many chemotherapy drugs. Although this is commonly mild and manageable with drugs such a loperamide, there are some notable exceptions. Irinotecan can cause severe and sometimes life-threatening diarrhoea. If this occurs within 24 hours after therapy and is associated with salivation and sweating, it is likely secondary to acute cholinergic syndrome. This is best managed with atropine in a specialist centre. Irinotecan-induced diarrhoea occurring days after therapy can also be severe and high-dose loperamide is often required. Diarrhoea may also occur in the context of neutropenia. Diarrhoea associated with fever and abdominal pain may indicate colonic infection and in particular typhlitis. This is a life-threatening infection of the large bowel wall, most commonly of the ascending colon, caused by Gram-negative bacteria, which requires intensive in-patient therapy with hydration and antibiotics.

Neurological toxicity

Neurological toxicity is a common feature of microtubule poisons such as the vinca alkaloids (e.g. vincristine), the taxanes (docetaxel and paclitaxel) and newer compunds such as eribulin. In addition, platinum salts used in chemotherapy regimens (cisplatin, carboplatin and oxaliplatin) frequently cause neuropathy during therapy. The commonest manifestation of chemotherapy-induced neurotoxicity is of peripheral sensory neuropathy in a stocking-and-glove distribution. This is frequently associated with loss of vibration sense, proprioception and deep-tendon reflexes, although these are rarely symptomatic. Although the symptoms of peripheral neuropathy can improve after discontinuation of therapy, residual symptoms many months or even years later are common. Cisplatin frequently causes irreversible ototoxicity, resulting in high-frequency deafness. As the nerve damage that induces these signs and symptoms of neurotoxicity results from cumulative drug dosing, awareness of symptoms and appropriate dose reduction or cessation are important steps in limiting toxicity and maintaining quality of life.

Motor neuropathy is much less common, especially in the absence of sensory symptoms. The exception is oxaliplatin-induced reversible acute cold aggravated neuropathy, most commonly presenting with pharyngeal spasm. Avoidance of cold drinks and cold environments for 2–4 hours after therapy significantly reduces the frequency of attacks. Autonomic neuropathy is most common with the vinca alkaloids, in particular vicristine. The commonest manifestation is constipation, and again the toxic effects are cumulative. Continued treatment can result in paralytic ileus, even with the appropriate use of laxatives.

Nausea and vomiting

Nausea and vomiting used to be the dose-limiting toxicity for the majority of chemotherapy drugs, induced through central action on the chemoreceptor trigger zone, but also through effects on the upper GI tract. However, the introduction of corticosteroids and $5HT_3$ (e.g. ondansetron) and neurokinin 1 (NK1) receptor antagonists (e.g. aprepitant) has significantly improved the tolerability of the commonly used agents. Patients will generally be given these anti-emetics as pre-medication and to take for 24–48 hours after chemotherapy to cover the 'acute' toxicity period. Additional 'breakthrough' antiemetics are frequently provided, with agents such as metocolopramide or cyclizine. 'Late' nausea and vomiting occurring 3–5 days after chemotherapy treatment is best managed with corticosteroids and metoclopramide. Although powerful against vomiting, the $5HT_3$ antagonists have their own side effect of constipation.

Late effects of chemotherapy

Over the last few decades, treatment of cancer has improved significantly, and more patients are becoming long-term survivors of the disease (see Chapter 18). This means that it has become more important to recognise the potential risks and identify the long-term effects of treatments, including chemotherapy.

Pulmonary toxicity

Chemotherapy-induced lung injury is increasingly recognised as a cause of respiratory symptoms in cancer patients, although it should be noted that progression of disease and respiratory tract infection (RTI) are significantly more common. Many classes of chemotherapy agent are implicated, including alkylating agents, antitumour antibiotics, antimetabolites and antimicrotubules. The exact mechanism of lung injury is poorly understood but likely involves epithelial and endothelial damage resulting in inflammatory cell infiltrates and subsequent fibrosis.

The symptoms of chemotherapy-induced lung injury can develop weeks, months or occasionally even years after treatment. Patients commonly complain of dyspnoea, malaise, fatigue and nonproductive cough. Clinical examination will often reveal bibasal crackles. Confirmation of the diagnosis can be difficult as radiological investigations may be normal. Chest x-ray (CXR) may show reticulonodular infiltrates, although high-resolution computed tomography (CT) will be significantly more sensitive. In addition, pulmonary function tests reveal a restrictive pattern and a reduction in transfer factor. Lung biopsy is the gold-standard investigation.

Treatment of chemotherapy-induced lung injury can be difficult and should involve specialist respiratory physicians. Withdrawal of the causative drug is necessary and corticosteriods may be useful. As the disease progresses, cough suppressants, calcium channel blockers to reduce pulmonary hypertension and narcotics to reduce distressing symptoms may be necessary.

The antitumour antibiotic bleomycin is used in the treatment of patients with testicular tumours, which is often highly curable; however, the development of pulmonary toxicity carries a high mortality. Thus, every care is taken in these patients to identify preexisting lung disease, and doses should not exceed 450–500 mg. If these patients do become unwell, the use of high-concentration oxygen should be avoided, as this increases the risk of pulmonary toxicity.

Cardiac toxicity

Many chemotherapeutic drugs produce toxic effects on the heart. The most important of these are the anthracyclines, although other agents have also been implicated, including antimicrotubule agents. Acute cardiac toxicity occurs within days and is associated with acute myocyte damage and myocarditis. Subacute damage develops more insidiously over months, with increasing fatigue, tachycardia and eventually pulmonary oedema and right-heart congestive symptoms. Chemotherapy-induced cardiac damage may not present for several years after treatment and is generally associated with a cardiomyopathy.

A number of comorbid conditions increase the risk of cardiac toxicity, including hypertension, previous ischaemic heart disease, uncontrolled arrhythmias and diabetes mellitus. In addition, it is well recognised that for certain agents there is a threshold dose above which cardiac toxicity becomes more frequent. Patients will rarely receive more than 450–500 mg/m^2 of doxorubicin or 900 mg/m^2 of epirubicin, as above these doses up to 30% of patients will suffer cardiac toxicity.

Treatment of chemotherapy-induced cardiomyopathy involves inotropic support and afterload reduction. The use of angiotensin-converting enzyme (ACE) inhibitors can stabilise the condition and reduce further deterioration. Beta blockers may also be useful.

Second cancers

It is well established that many anticancer treatments are associated with an increased risk of development of a second cancer. Development of second cancers is not always related to treatment and patients who have been previously treated for non-Hodgkin lymphoma, testicular tumours and paediatric malignancies are at increased risk of other non-treatment-related cancers.

The most common second malignancy related to chemotherapy treatment is leukaemia, particularly acute myeloid leukaemia, but also acute lymphoblastic leukaemia. In some series, the risk of developing these malignancies can be twofold increased and is associated with higher doses, higher dose intensity and longer duration of treatment.

Alkylating agents are commonly used in the treatment of many cancers and the risk of developing leukaemia begins to increase after 2 years, peaking approximately 5–10 years after treatment. Leukaemia that develops following alkylating agents tends to exhibit specific genetic mutations and can be difficult to treat, with a poor prognosis.

Other chemotherapy agents, such as topoisomerase II inhibitors (e.g. etoposide), can also increase the risk of leukaemia. This differs from that caused by alkylating agents in that it tends to occur earlier, peaking at 2 years. In addition, it also responds better to treatment and has a better prognosis.

Other types of cancer have been linked to chemotherapy, such as bladder cancer, linked to high doses of cyclophosphamide.

Fertility

Chemotherapy can result in impairment of fertility, and the effects will be dependent on the drugs, the dose (cumulative dose) and the gender and age of the patient. Most chemotherapy regimens are combinations, and these are more gonadotoxic than single agents, with alkylating agents such as cyclophosphamide being the most gonadotoxic. Little information is available on the effects on fertility of some of the newer agents, such as taxanes. The germinal epithelium and testes primordial sperm cells are very sensitive to cytotoxic chemotherapy and treatment will result in a very profound and quick drop in spermatogenesis, reflected in a reduction in the sperm count. Certain agents produce only a temporary reduction in sperm counts, such as vinca alkloids and anthracylines, while others result in a prolonged period of azoospermia; these include cyclophosphamide and cisplatin. The Leydig cells, which produce testosterone, are generally more chemoresistant than the germinal epithelium, and while mild Leydig cell impairment can occur, the clinical significance of this is unclear.

In females, cyctotoxic treatment reduces the pool of oocytes. Given the pool is fixed at birth, the effect of such treatment will be age-dependant. The risk of amenorrohea and of treatment-induced menopause is known to be low (<20%) in women who are receiving adjuvant chemotherapy for breast cancer and are under 30 years of age, although menses may become irregular. The risk is also low in non-alkylating regimens used for Hodgkin lymphoma. However, in women over the age of 40 years treated with chemotherapy for breast cancer or for Hodgkin lymphoma with a procarbazine-containing regimen, the risk of induced menopause is high (>80%). Other regimens are associated with a very high risk of amenorrohea. The effects of chemotherapy on fertility may be compounded by the disease itself, as well as by the surgical and/or radiotherapy treatment required.

In terms of fertility preservation prior to commencing treatment, women with a partner or donor sperm may consider embryo cryopreservation, which involves a cycle of *in vitro* fertilisation (IVF). This has potential problems in terms of delaying systemic treatment. In breast cancer which is oestrogen receptor (ER) positive, the impact of ovarian stimulation with elevated oestrogen levels (necessary to release ova) is uncertain. Although IVF is not a risk factor for breast cancer in the general population, its effect in women who have had breast cancer is not yet the subject of sufficient data. For women without a partner, egg harvesting and cryopreservation may be an option, although this still involves ovarian stimulation. The preservation of a small piece of ovarian tissue or of an entire ovary (ovarian tissue cryopreservation) can also be considered, but its efficacy is not well established. It may also be considered to minimise delays and/or avoid ovarian stimulation The use of gonadotrophin-releasing hormone (GnRH) analogues such as goserelin with chemotherapy to 'rest' the ovaries and allow resumption of normal ovarian function is an option that can be considered. Sperm banking is a highly successful technique for fertility preservation in men.

Further reading

DeVita, V.T., Lawrence, T.S., Rosenberg, S.A., Weinberg, R.A. & DePinho, R.A. (eds) (2008) *DeVita, Hellman, and Rosenberg's Cancer: Principles & Practice of Oncology*, 8th edn. Lippincott Williams & Wilkins, Philadelphia.

European Organisation for Research and Treatment of Cancer (1994, 1999, 2006, 2009) Common toxicity criteria (CTC), http://www.eortc.org/documentation-and-references/common-toxicity-criteria-ctc (last accessed 8 March 2013).

LIVESTRONG: Fertile Hope Web site, www.fertilehope.org.

My New Hair Web site, www.mynewhair.org.

National Health Service (2011) Guidelines for the management of chemotherapy and systemic anticancer therapy induced toxicities within primary care (adult solid tumour oncology and adult haemato-oncology), http://www.lpc-online.org.uk/bkpage/files/175/necn_guidelines_for_community_management_of_chemotherapy_toxicity_v1.2.pdf (last accessed 8 March 2013).

CHAPTER 7

Radiotherapy

Alastair Thomson[1] and Mark Beresford[2]

[1]Royal Cornwall Hospital (Sunrise Centre), Truro, Cornwall, UK
[2]Royal United Hospital, Bath, UK

OVERVIEW

- Radiotherapy is the delivery of focussed high-energy x-rays in order to damage cancer cells
- A course of radiotherapy involves a planning appointment followed by a number of daily treatment visits
- Differences in the biology of cancer cells and normal cells are exploited to maximise tumour kill and minimise side effects
- Some types of cancer are more radiosensitive than others
- Oncology emergencies such as spinal cord compression and superior vena caval obstruction can be effectively managed with radiotherapy

---

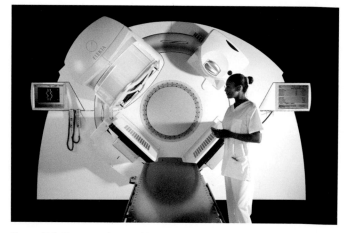

Figure 7.1 Linear accelerator (LinAc). This modern LinAc has onboard CT capabilities, allowing it to image the patient at the same time as delivering treatment. The computer screen on the left shows the position of the multileaf collimator shielding, while the screen on the right controls the position and rotation of the bed and treatment machine.

Introduction

Radiotherapy is the most effective nonsurgical treatment for malignant disease. It involves the delivery of high-energy x-ray beams targeted at the cancer. The x-rays damage DNA, leading to cell death.

When radiotherapy was first developed, it used the radiation naturally emitted by decaying isotopes (e.g. Cobalt[60]). Today the most common form of radiotherapy utilises photons generated by a linear accelerator (usually shortened to LinAc), a machine which uses electricity to fire electrons across a vacuum (Figure 7.1). When the electrons hit a target at the head of the LinAc, photon radiation is released and focussed (collimated) towards a particular point. The beams can be modified by multileaf collimators (fingerlike tungsten shielding which moves in and out of the treatment aperture) to allow conformal shaping of the treatment fields. The energy of the photon beams can be altered, with higher-energy beams being able to penetrate deeper into the patient.

Treatment practicalities

Radiotherapy is a targeted treatment. At a first appointment (usually called a simulation or planning visit) the oncologist will define the tumour target using either x-ray imaging or, for more precise definition, a dedicated computed tomography (CT) or magnetic resonance imaging (MRI) scan in the treatment position. Critical normal structures near to the radiotherapy field are identified and defined as organs at risk such that they can be kept within a maximum safe dose (Figure 7.2).

Radiotherapy treatment doses are generally fractionated into a number of smaller daily doses; the number depends on the treatment intent and the type of cancer being treated. Treatments with curative intent are typically delivered with three or four beams daily, each taking a few minutes. The overall treatment time depends on the complexity of individual treatment plans, but is typically 15–20 minutes, much of which involves ensuring the patient is in the correct position. The treatment is invisible and painless but the patient must lie still and be compliant as the radiographers leave the room for delivery.

Accurate positioning is crucial to ensuring that the treatment delivered matches the plan designed. Patients are marked with small permanent tattoos on the skin, which are lined up with treatment room lasers to ensure that no rotational movement takes place on the treatment couch. To ensure positioning is stable and reproducible, bespoke vacuum-moulded polystyrene bead bags,

ABC of Cancer Care, First Edition.
Edited by Carlo Palmieri, Esther Bird and Richard Simcock.
© 2013 John Wiley & Sons, Ltd. Published 2013 by John Wiley & Sons, Ltd.

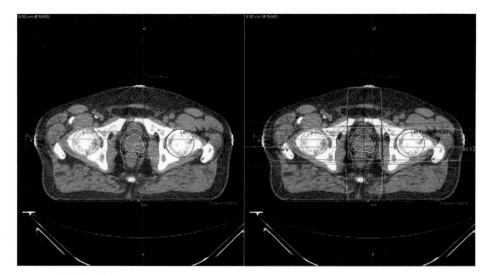

Figure 7.2 CT plan of prostate radiotherapy volumes. The yellow outline demarcates the prostate target volume (with an additional margin added to account for subclinical disease and organ movement). Organs at risk include the bladder (dark blue) and rectum (brown). The image on the right includes the radiotherapy beams and dose contours.

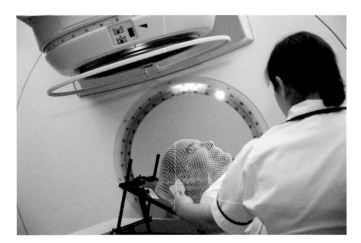

Figure 7.3 Patient receiving radiotherapy for a brain tumour immobilised in a thermoplastic shell (or 'mask'), which is fixed to the treatment couch underneath the linear accelerator. The radiographer is checking the accuracy of the setup using positional lasers mounted in the room's walls.

limb supports or Perspex shells can be used. Thermoplastic masks are created for brain and head and neck cancer treatments, to ensure millimetre accuracy (Figure 7.3). Accuracy of treatment is verified by x-ray or cone-beam CT images taken throughout the course of treatment, to ensure that anatomic landmarks match up with those on the initial planning scans.

The dose of radiotherapy is expressed in Gray (Gy) – a measure of absorbed dose at the target.

Radiobiological principles

The energy of radiotherapy damages the DNA of a cell, either directly or indirectly by interaction with oxygen to form free radicals. When a cell is damaged by radiotherapy it may undergo immediate cell death through apoptosis (lethal damage) or it may be able to repair itself (sublethal damage). Tumour cells have deficient cell repair and are less able to recover from sublethal damage. It is this difference between normal and malignant cells

that is exploited by fractionating radiotherapy, over a number of days or weeks. Multiple sequential sublethal doses preferentially damage cancer, leading eventual cell death. Over a course of therapy, cancer cells will continue to grow (repopulate). If the fractionation is over too long a period, the cancer's repopulation will reduce its effect. Attempts have been made to reduce the overall treatment time in some tumour types, such as lung and head and neck cancer, by treating patients twice a day. This has radiobiological advantages in reducing repopulation of cancer cells, but it does result in more acute side effects, and patients have to be carefully supported. Radiotherapy will inevitably cause some degree of damage to normal tissues (see Chapter 9). Some tissues and tumours are more sensitive to radiotherapy than others (see Table 7.1). Normal tissue damage is reduced by shielding and by highly conformal techniques using advanced computer algorithms to 'shape' the radiotherapy treatment to the cancer.

External factors can influence the effect of radiotherapy. Good oxygenation of tissue is required for maximum effect, so maintaining adequate haemoglobin levels is important for some tumour types. Concurrent chemotherapy administration can potentiate the effects of radiotherapy cell damage and improve outcomes, but may also increase toxicity.

Table 7.1 Radiosensitivity of different tumour types.

Degree of radiosensitivity	Effect of radiotherapy	Tumour types
High	Curable with radiotherapy alone	Lymphoma, germ cell tumours
Moderate	May be curable with high doses of radiotherapy (perhaps as adjunct to surgery or with chemotherapy)	Squamous cell carcinomas (lung, head and neck, cervix, skin) Breast, colorectal, prostate, bladder
Low	Radiotherapy less effective and mainly restricted to palliative use	Melanoma, kidney

Treatment intent

Radiotherapy can be used with curative intent, or to palliate symptoms from the tumour. The aims of the treatment will be individualised and depend on the following:

- *Tumour factors*: How advanced is the tumour and how sensitive is it to irradiation (see Table 7.1)?
- *Treatment factors*: How large is the volume of radiotherapy required to cover all the tumour, and how close is it to sensitive normal tissues that will limit the dose?
- *Patient factors*: Are there medical comorbidities which increase potential for side effects? Is the patient willing and of sufficiently good health to tolerate a more intense course of radiotherapy?

Palliative radiotherapy

Irradiation is a useful modality by which to palliate cancer symptoms. Palliative treatments are usually delivered in short courses or single fractions, in order to reduce patient travel and inconvenience. These large doses given over short periods can cause late side effects and therefore would not be appropriate in curative treatment courses. Typical indications include symptomatic bone metastases (where radiotherapy achieves significant pain relief in approximately half of patients), multiple brain metastases and where the reduction of pain or bleeding from an advanced tumour is desired.

Emergency radiotherapy

Radiotherapy is important in the treatment of the oncological emergencies of superior vena cava obstruction (SVCO) and spinal cord compression (see Chapter 13).

Radical radiotherapy

Radiotherapy can be used with curative intent by itself, for example in skin or head and neck cancers. It can also be used as part of multimodality treatment. Examples include in the neoadjuvant setting (as the initial part of treatment) in locally advanced rectal cancer before surgery and in the adjuvant setting (after surgery to reduce the risk of relapse) in breast cancer. Radiotherapy effect may be potentiated by giving it in combination with chemotherapy (e.g. in cervical and oesophageal cancers).

Longer courses are generally used, with convergence of several radiotherapy beams on to the target volume from different angles in order to maximise tumour control probability and limit normal tissue side effects. Stereotactic radiotherapy uses even more beams to enhance this targeting and shaping of the irradiation, and is used in treating solitary or oligometastatic disease in the brain (see Chapter 4). Stereotactic radiosurgery can be used in the radical treatment of lung cancer.

Brachytherapy is a technique in which radioactive sources are placed close to (intracavitary) or inside (interstitial) tumours. This gives a high dose of radiotherapy around the sources thus placed, but the dose falls off quickly with distance, leading to less irritation of the surrounding normal tissues. High-dose-rate (HDR) brachytherapy uses a highly active radioactive source, which is employed and then removed. This has the advantage of reducing toxicity and shortening treatment time, but comes with the problems of source insertion, anaesthetic and discomfort. Some prostate and gynaecological cancers are suitable for this approach. Low-dose-rate (LDR) brachytherapy uses slowly decaying radioactive sources permanently inserted into the tumour. Radioactive seed implants in early prostate cancer are the most prevalent example.

Intraoperative radiotherapy

The development of smaller radiotherapy machines has made it practical to consider the use of radiation at the time of surgery in the operating theatre. The greatest experience of this comes from the treatment of early breast cancer, where after removal of the tumour the treating team can deliver a dose of radiotherapy immediately to the tumour bed or insert a balloon into the cavity to allow the prompt treatment of the area by high-dose brachytherapy. Several large trials comparing this approach to standard external beam radiotherapy are underway around the world.

Intensity-modulated radiotherapy and image-guided radiotherapy

Intensity-modulated radiotherapy (IMRT) uses powerful computerised treatment planning systems to design highly complex radiotherapy plans. Rather than using three or four treatment beams, these plans will often use eight or more, with each beam composed of multiple small segments. This has the effect of building dose profiles that can more flexibly cover the target while at the same time avoiding critical normal tissues. The technique is more resource intensive in the time taken to design and check treatment plans. IMRT has been proven to reduce long-term toxicity of treatment (e.g. the salivary gland damage caused by head and neck radiotherapy).

While some tumour targets will be immobile (e.g. bone tumours), some targets will move (e.g. lung tumours with respiration, prostate tumours with rectal and bladder filling). Image-guided radiotherapy (IGRT) uses imaging technology (usually cone-beam CT) mounted on the LinAc. Images are collected during treatment to assess the motion of relevant structures and to provide small shifts in the position of the treatment beam. This ensures accuracy but also reduces the need to add large 'safety margins' to treatment plans and therefore reduces normal tissue radiation.

New technologies

Radiotherapy technology continues to advance with the development in computer processor power, allowing for increasingly complex planning algorithms. Treatments may now be delivered by dynamic arc techniques, where the dose is delivered by multiple beamlets as the machine rotates around the patient. In addition, developments in hardware, including robotic LinAcs (e.g. Cyberknife™), are increasing the flexibility of treatment machines. These advances are combining improved diagnostic imaging (fusing planning images with MRI and positron emission technology

(PET) images) and improved targeting of radiotherapy (tracking targets during treatments to account for organ motion).

Investment in radiotherapy is permitting the construction of proton units. These treatment units (each the size of a football field) produce high-energy particles that penetrate deeply into tissues but stop at a defined depth. This allows for high-dose treatment to deep-seated tumours without causing critical damage to vital organs, for example in the treatment of brain tumours.

In addition to these physical and technical developments, there are many research programmes which combine radiotherapy with drugs, including chemotherapies and newer biological therapies (e.g. the use of the monoclonal antibody cetuximab during head and neck radiotherapy).

Further reading

Ajithkumar, T.V. & Hatcher, H.M. (2011) *Specialist Training in Oncology*. Mosby Elsevier, Missouri.

Hoskin, P. (2007) *Radiotherapy in Practice: External Beam Radiotherapy*. OUP, Oxford.MyRadiotherapy.com, www.myradiotherapy.com

Royal College of Radiologists virtual radiotherapy department, www.goingfora.com.

CHAPTER 8

Toxicities of Radiotherapy

Russell Burcombe[1], Jonathan Hicks[2], and Richard Simcock[3]

[1]Kent Oncology Centre, Maidstone Hospital, Maidstone, Kent, UK
[2]Beatson West of Scotland Cancer Centre, Glasgow, UK
[3]Sussex Cancer Centre, Royal Sussex County Hospital, Brighton, UK

OVERVIEW

- Radiation causes side effects locally in the tissues being irradiated
- Acute side effects are short lived and caused by damage to cells with rapid turnover
- Late side effects have different causes, may appear many years later and may be permanent
- Side effects may require specialist input and management
- Previously seen severe toxicities (such as brachial plexopathy) can now be avoided with modern targeted radiotherapy techniques

---

Introduction

Radiation damage to DNA kills cancer cells but also harms normal tissues.

Most normal tissues are able to repair DNA breaks, though the temporary damage from radiotherapy causes side effects. Most side effects are short lived, but some may be permanent. The timing of radiation side effects relates to the speed of cell turnover; thus, rapidly dividing cells (e.g. oral mucosa) show damage quickly, while slow-growing cells (e.g. neurones) may manifest toxicity long after radiation is complete.

A sigmoid dose–response relationship exists between radiation dose, tumour cell kill and normal tissue damage. Tumour cells are more sensitive to radiation than normal tissues. Higher radiation doses increase the probability of eradicating tumours to secure permanent local control, but at the cost of greater normal tissue damage. Oncologists exploit this therapeutic window by delivering a sufficient radiation dose to sterilise tumour cells but minimise permanent side effects.

Radiation sensitivity

Radiation sensitivity varies between individuals. Patients with rare DNA damage repair defects exhibit acute severe and late hypersensitivity to therapeutic radiation. At present, no sufficiently sensitive

assays that can predict radiation sensitivity are available for use in routine clinical practice.

Acute side effects

Acute side effects occur during or a few weeks after treatment and are caused by direct cytotoxicity to rapidly growing normal cells. The effects are usually short lived and preferentially affect rapidly growing cells, such as bone marrow, skin and mucous membranes.

Late side effects

Late side effects occur weeks to months after treatment and their aetiology remains contentious. Effects may be permanent. Mechanisms include acute damage to blood vessels, causing late tissue damage. Depletion of normal stem cells that are slow to regenerate may also contribute to late side effects.

The side effects of radiotherapy depend on the area being treated.

Skin

Skin reactions begin about a week after starting treatment and usually peak in severity about a week after radiotherapy is complete. Most patients suffer skin erythema. Some patients develop peeling (desquamation) of the skin as dose accumulates (see Figure 8.1).

The severity of skin reactions can be affected by both the total radiation dose and the individual daily (fraction) dose. Concurrent drug treatment may also increase the severity of reaction. Reactions are often worse in skin folds in the treatment area (e.g. inframammary fold, groin).

Patients are advised to avoid friction (from tightly fitted clothes or towels), chemical irritants (perfumes, powders or deodorants), razor blades and excessive heat or cold during treatment. Bathing or showering with warm water and a mild soap is allowed, but any oils or lotions are discouraged.

Hydrocortisone (1%) can ease the itching some patients experience and aqueous cream, hydrophilic moisturisers or aloe vera gels are effective against dry erythema.

Moist desquamation is best treated in a specialist radiotherapy centre: hydrocolloid or alginate dressings, silver sulfadiazine lyofoam, Mepilex® or Melonin are recommended.

Severe acute skin radiation reactions take 2–6 weeks to resolve, but recovery is usually complete.

ABC of Cancer Care, First Edition.
Edited by Carlo Palmieri, Esther Bird and Richard Simcock.

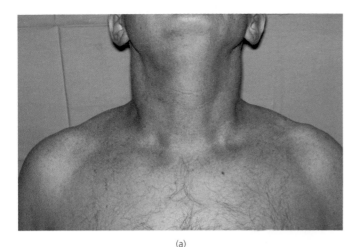

(a)

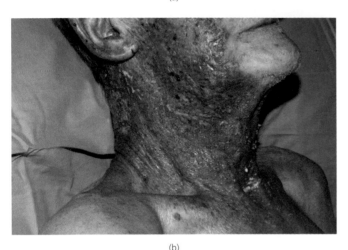

(b)

Figure 8.1 Skin of a patient receiving adjuvant radiotherapy for a head and neck cancer at the end of a course of treatment, with the reddened (erythematous) skin clearly shown in the irradiated area. In (a) the reaction is very mild, with only minimal erythema, but in (b) the reaction is severe, with desquamation and subsequent crusting of the skin. It is not known why different patients will have different levels of normal tissue reaction to the same treatment.

Bone marrow suppression

The vertebrae, sternum and pelvis contain all of an adult's active bone marrow. Irradiating these sites can lead to bone marrow suppression. This can be accentuated if chemotherapy is given concurrently.

Fatigue

Tiredness is a common symptom. Severity varies between individuals. The aetiology is unknown. Maintaining physical fitness, or regular exercise, even to a low level, can counteract fatigue.

Methylphenidate or Modafinil 200 mg can be used to treat fatigue and may have some benefit on cognitive functioning and depression, although it can cause anxiety and insomnia.

Brain

Radiotherapy to the brain will cause alopecia. In contrast to the alopecia caused by chemotherapy (see Chapter 6), hair regrowth can be extremely slow and often incomplete due to damage to hair follicles. The extent of hair loss (and recovery) depends on the dose of radiotherapy, with permanent loss at higher doses. Alopecia starts 2–3 weeks into treatment, with regrowth typical at 6 months.

Radiation to the brain can cause nausea, headache and effects on memory and concentration. This occurs through a combination of vascular damage and demyelination. Whole-brain radiotherapy can lead to profound and debilitating tiredness, which can cause significant functional impairment ('somnolence syndrome'). The fatigue is mild or moderate starting 2–3 weeks after first radiotherapy dose but may persist for a number of months and does not improve with rest.

Fatigue is typically more profound than the more feared effect on memory and concentration. The timing and severity of cognitive dysfunction after cerebral radiation remains poorly understood.

Simple analgesics, antiemetics and steroids can be given as required and dosed according to symptoms.

Moist desquamation both behind the ears and in the external auditory canals may develop. Hearing can be impaired both in the short term through development of a reactive otitis media and in the longer term by direct ototoxicity at the level of the cochlea.

The brain may experience reactive oedema, which should be treated with reducing doses of steroids. Steroid toxicities (glucose intolerance, proximal myopathy, sleep disturbance) are frequent and the therapy should be closely monitored. Some patients receiving palliative whole brain radiotherapy may become steroid dependent but efforts should be made to titrate down to the lowest possible dose.

Head and neck

Because of the sensitivity of the oral mucosa and its important roles in nutrition, digestion and taste acute side effects during head and neck radiotherapy are debilitating and require regular specialist review (see Box 8.1).

Box 8.1 **Oral care during radiotherapy**

- If possible, carry out dental assessment prior to treatment, with optimisation of dental plaque removal and control of periodontal infection: dental hygienist and chlorhexidine.
- Encourage frequent mouth cleaning: sterile water, 1 tsp. of salt in 1 l water or 1–2 tsp. of baking soda in 1 l water.
- Avoid alcohol containing rinses during treatment.
- Use tooth sponges and baby toothbrush for oral hygiene.
- Use anti-inflammatory mouthwashes (e.g. Difflam®).
- Ensure patients receive adequate analgesia, topical and systemic: liquid morphine may be necessary to control the pain of severe mucositis.
- Patients with dentures are at an increased risk of mucositis due to trauma leading to mucosal injury and infection.
- Candidiasis is common and exacerbates mucositis: topical nystatin 1 ml q.d.s. is effective, but compliance may be an issue. The use of systemic antifungals in addition is appropriate: Fluconazole 50–100 mg.
- Use oral Caphosol™ mouthwash.

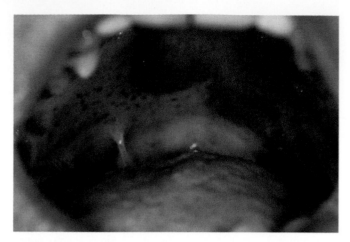

Figure 8.2 Mucositis, showing the oral cavity in a patient receiving radical radiotherapy. Sloughing and ulceration of the mucosa is seen in the left tonsillar area, with painful reddened mucosa on the left side. This is often misdiagnosed as candidiasis.

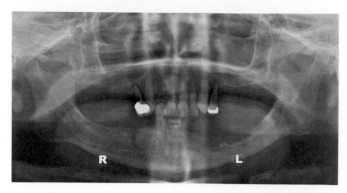

Figure 8.3 Orthopantogram showing osteoradionecrosis causing destruction of the lower left mandible and upper right maxilla in a patient previously treated with curative radiotherapy for a head and neck cancer.

Oral mucositis

As with skin, the severity of reaction of the mucus membranes depends on radiation dose and fractionation. It follows a similar time course from 2 weeks into radiotherapy up to 6 weeks after completion. Mucositis occurs due to the death of the basal cells of the oral mucosal epithelium. Initial erythema and tenderness fades to a pale membrane, which can evolve into ulceration (see Figure 8.2). This mucosa is then predisposed to superadded fungal infection. Zinc supplementation (zinc sulphate 220 mg b.d.) can reduce the severity of mucositis.

Oral care and hygiene (see Box 8.1) requires careful attention during radiotherapy as severe mucositis may prevent completion of the prescribed course of radiation.

Dry mouth (xerostomia)

Irradiation of the salivary glands (parotid or submandibular) can lead to permanent dry mouth. Xerostomia can start within a week of commencing radiotherapy, with initial thick viscous saliva giving way to a dry mouth. Long-term xerostomia may be relieved by artificial saliva sprays and gels. Pilocarpine Hydrocarpine tablets (5 mg t.d.s. with meals) can help, but causes severe sweating. Acupuncture has also shown benefit in clinical trials (see Chapter 15).

In addition, the mouth may be affected by fissuring at the corners (angular stomatitis), tongue atrophy and painful dentures. These problems exacerbate issues with sleep, speech and daily comfort.

Taste loss occurs quickly during radiotherapy, but in most cases normal taste returns after 2–3 months.

Late radiation effects on the blood supply of the mandible can be disastrous. If teeth are removed (dental decay is rapid in a mouth affected by radiation xerostomia) and the healing socket becomes infected, the jaw can break down and die (osteoradionecrosis). This condition requires long-term management by maxillofacial surgery (see Figure 8.3).

Chest

In the thorax, most side effects arise from oesophageal and lung irradiation.

Oesophagitis

Acute oesophagitis results from thinning of the squamous epithelial layer; subsequent late effects may disrupt swallowing by either stricture or functional compromise through nerve damage. Initially pain on swallowing (odynophagia) occurs, but this is then replaced by dysphagia.

Oesophageal ulceration is rare but can occur.

Patients require dietary modification (see Chapter 14) and symptom control. Acid suppression with proton pump inhibitors can be helpful and regular analgesia with liquid morphine (if required) has a systemic and topical effect. Oxcetocaine (a mixture of antacid and local anaesthetic) may be useful prior to eating. Promotility agents such as metoclopramide may help gastric transit.

Radiotherapy-induced stricture may require oesophageal dilatation. Swallowing dysfunction can lead to aspiration pneumonia, may require advice from the speech and language team and very occasionally necessitates long-term nasogastric feeding.

Pneumonitis

Acute lung inflammation (pneumonitis) can occur 1–3 months after radiotherapy, presenting as cough and shortness of breath. There may be associated temperature and the condition is often misdiagnosed as infection.

Treatment is only required if breathlessness is severe as it is usually self-limiting. Steroids (Dexamethasone 2–4 mg each morning) are prescribed for 2–6 weeks.

Chronic pulmonary fibrosis may produce characteristic radiological changes and loss of lung function. This is not reversible.

Smoking will increase both the acute and late effects of radiotherapy and all smokers should be offered support in quitting the habit.

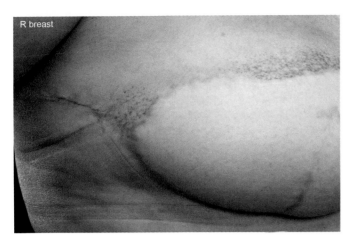

Figure 8.4 Reconstructed breast after mastectomy and radiotherapy. Telengiectasia in the irradiated skin can be seen in the scar line, contrasted with the normal unirradiated skin in the donor tissue of the reconstruction.

Breast

Postoperative breast or chest wall irradiation is commonly required after breast conserving surgery or mastectomy and forms a large percentage of the workload of any radiotherapy department. The skin of the breast develops typical acute reactions. Years after radiation (typically 4–5), skin telangiectasia and atrophy may arise due to dilatation of the vessels within a few millimetres of the epidermis. Late telangiectasia is more common after a severe acute inframammary moist desquamation skin reaction. Pulsed-dye laser treatment can be very effective against telengiectasia but several treatments may be required (see Figure 8.4).

Lymphoedema

Irradiation of the supraclavicular and axillary nodes may cause severe late toxicities. Damage to the lymphatic system can cause lymphoedema of the arm. The irreversible arm swelling can lead to profound disability in the affected limb. Lymphoedema is more common following extensive axillary surgery, post-operative axillary irradiation infection and obesity. Treatment is supportive, with manual lymph drainage, skin and nail care, compression bandaging and therapeutic exercise.

Irradiation of the supraclavicular area can lead to shoulder stiffness. In a previous era excess dose led to a painful syndrome of brachial plexopathy – fortunately now an exceptionally rare side effect.

Abdomen

Vomiting

Vomiting can occur within minutes or hours of radiotherapy to the stomach or after high doses of palliative radiotherapy to the spine. Patients should be given prophylactic 5HT3 antagonists (ondansetron, granesetron). Further antiemetics, including steroids, may be required (see Table 8.1).

Table 8.1 Managing gastrointestinal (GI) toxicity.

Symptom	Radiotherapy target	Treatment
Anorexia	A common symptom of any advanced cancer	Dietary advice (see Chapter 14) Low-dose steroid
Nausea and Vomiting	Lung Oesophagus Stomach Pelvis Thoracic and lumbar spine	Oral Domperidone 20 mg q.d.s. Oral Cyclizine 50 mg t.d.s. Levopromazine (Nozinan) 6.25 mg q.d.s. Buccastem Subcutaneous infusion over 24 hours Cyclizine 150 mg Levopromazine 25 mg
Diarrhoea	Pelvis Anorectal Cervix Prostate Palliative bone treatment (lumbar spine / pelvis)	Loperamide 4mg prn or codeine phosphate Low fat/low residue diet and avoidance of milk products NSAID anti-inflammatory drug Sulfasalazine 500mg bd. Oral sulcrafate (improves bowel function, but unpleasant to take)
Proctitis	Anorectal Cervix Prostate	Steroid enema or Proctofoam with cortisone Mesalazine used as an enema, delayed absorbing capsule or rectal suppository Sucralfate enemas; an aluminum hydroxide complex of sulfated sucrose nonsteroidal anti-inflammatory drugs (NSAIDs)

Lower abdomen

Change in bowel habit is common. Small bowel irradiation may induce a radiation enteritis. The timing depends on total dose, fractionation and the total volume of the bowel irradiated. After a large single fraction, enteritis may occur an hour following treatment; with longer courses of smaller fraction sizes symptoms may start 2–4 weeks into treatment. Stool frequency is higher and stools may be softer, often accompanied by colicky or wind pains. A diarrhoea syndrome may develop. Alongside watery faeces, there may be mucus or 'slime' from the bowel wall, accompanied by small amounts of blood (see Table 8.1).

Bladder

Acute cystitis is typically mild in the short term, but damage to the urothelium may manifest itself up to a year after treatment. In the long term, bladder contraction and telangectasia can lead to pain on passing urine, frequency and haematuria.

Urine infection should be excluded and a good fluid intake maintained. Alkalinisation of urine using sodium bicarbonate or potassium citrate may help cystitis symptoms; cranberry capsules sometimes help. Oxybutynin chloride (starting at 5 mg b.d.) may ease urinary spasm, and the alpha blockers tamsulosin and terazocin help relieve hesitancy. For patients leaking urine, ephedrine hydrochloride 15–60 mg t.d.s. can increase bladder outflow resistance.

Rectum

Along with diarrhoea, proctitis is an almost universal side effect of rectal radiation (see Table 8.1). Rectal bleeding at 12–18 months following radiotherapy occurs after telangiectasia forms within the rectal lining. At sigmoidoscopy, bleeding points can be treated with thermal coagulation or formalin application. Haemorrhoids are common and are treated with conventional haemorrhoid creams.

Female genital tract

Irradiation of the female genital tract may produce a painful mucositis. The principles of good skin care should be followed when the vulva and vagina are in the radiotherapy field. Excess sitz baths are discouraged, as excess moisture can lead to softened skin and maceration. Topical lidocaine gel 2% can provide useful local analgesia.

In the longer term, vaginal stenosis and vaginal dryness may lead to painful sex and psychosexual morbidity. Open discussion of these symptoms in a supportive environment is required (see Chapter 17). Vaginal dilators and lubricants are helpful in preventing and managing vaginal stenosis, and an early return to normal sexual activity once acute effects have settled is advised (abstinence can further predispose to vaginal shortening and fibrosis). Oestrogen creams may improve vaginal elasticity.

Ovarian failure can be a consequence of ovarian radiation for pelvic malignancy causing premature menopause and infertility (see Chapter 17).

Further reading

Cancer Research UK (n.d.) Side effects of radiotherapy, http://cancerhelp.cancerresearchuk.org/about-cancer/treatment/radiotherapy/follow-up/long-term-side-effects-of-radiotherapy (last accessed 8 March 2013).

Royal College of Radiologists UK (1995) Management of adverse effects following breast radiotherapy, http://www.rcr.ac.uk/docs/oncology/pdf/maher.pdf (last accessed 8 March 2013).

Royal College of Radiologists UK (2006) Radiotherapy dose-fractionation, http://www.rcr.ac.uk/docs/oncology/pdf/dose-fractionation_final.pdf (last accessed 8 March 2013).

CHAPTER 9

Endocrine Therapy

Carlo Palmieri[1], Matthew Flook[2], and Duncan C. Gilbert[3]

[1]University of Liverpool, Department of Molecular and Clinical Cancer Medicine, The Royal Liverpool University Hospital & The Clatterbridge Cancer Centre, Liverpool, UK
[2]Imperial College Healthcare NHS Trust, London, UK
[3]Sussex Cancer Centre, Royal Sussex County Hospital, Brighton, UK

OVERVIEW

- Breast and prostate cancer are driven by the sex hormones oestrogen and testosterone respectively
- Endocrine therapy is a treatment which modulates and blocks the action of oestrogen and testosterone in cancer cells
- There are a number of endocrine therapies that can be used in breast and prostate cancer; the sequential use of these in advanced disease can delay the need for chemotherapy
- A limiting factor of endocrine therapy is the development of resistance
- 70% of breast cancers are oestrogen receptor positive and therefore amenable to endocrine therapy
- Endocrine therapy in the treatment of early-stage breast cancer improves overall survival
- In metastatic/advanced breast cancer, sequential endocrine therapy is the treatment of choice where possible and can delay the need for chemotherapy
- Targeted agents (trastuzumab, lapatinib and everolimus) can be used with endocrine therapy
- Androgen deprivation therapy (ADT) is of proven benefit when added to external-beam radiotherapy in the treatment of high-risk localised prostate cancers, and forms the backbone of the treatment of metastatic disease
- Prostate cancers require testosterone even at stages of disease previously thought to be hormone insensitive
- New drugs targeting testosterone synthesis and signalling have recently been introduced

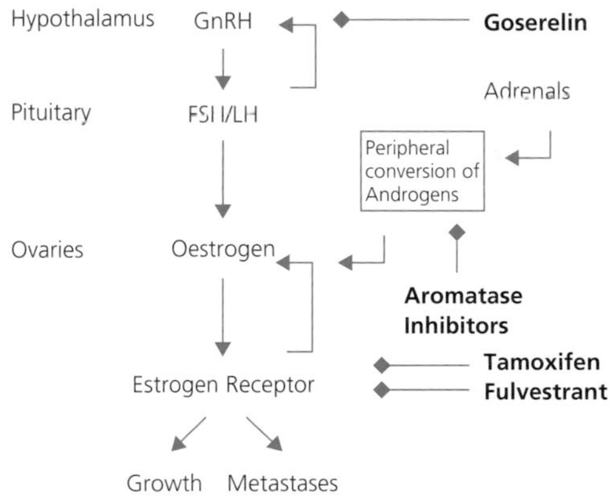

Figure 9.1 Schematic representation of the female hypothalamo-pituitary-gonadal axis, with drugs annotated.

Breast cancer

70% of breast cancers are oestrogen receptor (ER) positive, and for these cancers endocrine therapy is an important treatment in both the early and the advanced setting. In premenopausal women, the majority of oestrogen production is from the ovarian follicles. Following stimulation by gonadotrophin releasing hormone (GnRH) (also known as luteinising hormone-releasing hormone, LHRH) produced in the hypothalamus, the anterior pituitary gland produces luteinising hormone (LH) and follicle-stimulating hormone (FSH). LH stimulates thecal cells to synthesise androgens, while FSH stimulates granulosa cells to produce the enzyme aromatase enzyme, which then converts testosterone and androstenedione to oestradiol and oestrone respectively, in a process known as aromatisation (Figure 9.1). Oestrogen can also be produced peripherally in the liver, adrenal glands and adipose tissue via aromatisation, and it is these peripheral sources that are the key sites of oestrogen production in postmenopausal women. Oestrogen exerts its effect via binding to the endoplasmic reticulum, which in turn directly regulates the transcription of genes via its ability to bind to DNA. Endocrine therapy is aimed at modulating and disrupting this process by either blocking pituitary production of LH/FSH, blocking/degrading ER or inhibiting the peripheral production of oestradiol (Table 9.1). The menopausal status of the patient will determine the potential endocrine treatment options available.

Current endocrine therapy

Classes of endocrine agents and mechanisms of action are summarised in Table 9.1. All are oral medications, with the exception of fulvestrant, an intramuscular injection, and gonadotrophin-releasing hormone agonists (GnRHa), which are given as subcutaneous injections; both are given monthly.

ABC of Cancer Care, First Edition.
Edited by Carlo Palmieri, Esther Bird and Richard Simcock.
© 2013 John Wiley & Sons, Ltd. Published 2013 by John Wiley & Sons, Ltd.

Table 9.1 Classes of endocrine therapy agents, mechanisms of action and licensed agents currently available. 'Postmenopausal' means natural, surgically induced via oophrectomy or involving the use of LHRH agonist.

Endocrine therapy agent	Mechanism of action	Agent	Use
Selective oestrogen receptor modulator (SERM)	Inhibits and antagonises ER in breast cancer	Tamoxifen	Pre- and postmenopausal Early and advanced disease
Aromatase inhibitors	Inhibits aromatase and therefore peripheral production of oestradiol	*Nonsteriodal* • Anastrozole • Letrozole *Steriodal* • Exemestane	Postmenopausal Early and advanced disease
Selective oestrogen receptor downregulator (SERD)	Increases turnover of ER and therefore reduces levels	Fulvestrant	Postmenopausal Advanced disease
Ovarian ablation: • Gonadotrophin-releasing hormone agonist (GnRHa) • Oophrectomy • Radiotherapy	Causes downregulation of GnRH receptors in the pituitary gland and reduction in LH	Leuprolin Goserelin	Pre- and postmenopausal Early and advanced disease
Testosterone antagonist	Inhibits testosterone-binding androgen receptor (AR)	Cyproterone acetate Bicalutamide Enzalutamide	Prevents tumour flare with GnRH analogues Treats hot flushes (cyproterone) Maximal androgen blockade (bicalutamide) Advanced disease (enzalutamide)
Gonadotrophin-releasing hormone agonist (GnRHa)	Causes downregulation of GnRH receptors in the pituitary gland and reduction in LH	Leuprolin Goserelin	Localised disease (with radiotherapy) Long-term ADT in advanced disease
Steroids	Negative feedback on adrenal synthesis of testosterone	Dexamethasone	Castration refractory disease
CYP17 inhibitor	Inhibits testosterone synthesis	Abiraterone	Castration refractory disease

Adjuvant endocrine therapy

In early breast cancer, adjuvant endocrine therapy should be considered for all patients with ER-positive and/or progesterone-positive breast cancer, in order to reduce the risk of recurrence and death from the disease. There are no absolute contraindications to endocrine therapy, although individual agents may need to be avoided depending on comorbidities and risk factors.

In premenopausal patients, 5 years of treatment with tamoxifen is currently considered standard. However, ovarian suppression therapy in the form of ovarian ablation (surgical or GnRHa) can be considered, either alone (normally for 2–3 years) or in combination with tamoxifen or an aromatase inhibitor (AI). With regard to postmenopausal breast cancer, the therapeutic options include 5 years of tamoxifen or AI alone or a sequence of AI followed by tamoxifen (or the reverse) for a total of 5 years. The regimen selected will depend in part on the risk of relapse and comorbidities. Current guidance is that postmenopausal women should be exposed to an AI at some point during their adjuvant treatment. Recent data has shown 10 years of tamoxifen to significantly improve outcome as compared to 5 years of tamoxifen. Based on this data a discussion regarding the potential benefits and risks of extended tamoxifen treatment is reasonable in women who have completed 5 years of tamoxifen, and for whom an AI is not appropriate for example women remaining pre-menopausal.

The benefits of adjuvant tamoxifen therapy have been shown by the Early Breast Cancer Trialists' Collaborative Group (EBCTC); their data show that at 15 years there is a reduction in breast cancer-specific mortality, from 33.1 to 23.9% (a 9.2% absolute benefit), with 5 years of adjuvant tamoxifen (Figure 9.2). The same meta-analysis group has also demonstrated the benefits of ovarian

ablation and AI. These data support the importance of adjuvant endocrine therapy in early breast cancer.

Metastatic/advanced disease

In metastatic disease, endocrine therapy is an important treatment modality given its ease of administration and preferable toxicity profile compared to chemotherapy. The use of endocrine therapy is limited by the development of resistance to these agents. Patients with disease limited to bone or with low-volume visceral disease that is relatively asymptomatic are ideal candidates for endocrine therapy. Generally, endocrine therapy is used in a sequential manner, and the agent used will depend on the prior therapies chosen in the adjuvant setting. Given a lack of cross-resistance between steroidal and nonsteroidal AI, both classes can be used in sequence in the advanced disease setting.

Postmenopausal women

In women with no prior endocrine treatment or prior adjuvant tamoxifen, sequential use of a nonsteroidal AI (e.g. letrozole) followed by the steroidal AI exemestane and then fulvestrant is considered standard. With the introduction of adjuvant AIs, the optimal sequence of endocrine therapy will need redefining. Depending on the time between last exposure to the AI and disease recurrence, consideration will be between use of an AI from the other class or an alternative class of endocrine agent.

Premenopausal women

In premenopausal women, options include tamoxifen, ovarian ablation alone and ovarian ablation in combination with tamoxifen

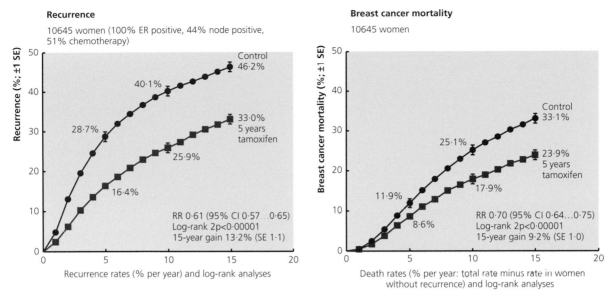

Figure 9.2 Effect of 5 years of adjuvant tamoxifen on disease recurrence and breast cancer mortality for ER Positive Disease. Reprinted from The Lancet, 2005; 365: 1687–1717, Early Breast Cancer Trialists' Collaborative Group (EBCTCG). Effects of chemotherapy and hormonal therapy for early breast cancer on recurrence and 15-year survival: an overview of the randomised trials. Copyright 2005, with permission from Elsevier.

or an AI. As first-line therapy, ovarian ablation (normally GnRHa) plus tamoxifen is considered standard.

Neoadjuvant setting

Endocrine therapy is a valuable treatment in those patients who have breast cancer in which surgery is not possible due to comorbidities or the size or nature of the disease. In such cases, primary or neoadjuvant endocrine therapy is a valuable treatment. Letrozole is considered the gold standard for postmenopausal women; for premenopausal women, GnRHa should be considered.

Male breast cancer

Male breast cancer is more commonly ER-positive than female breast cancer. However, given its rarity, few studies have been performed, and clinical decision making in male breast cancer has historically been extrapolated from studies in women. Tamoxifen is the established standard, with several retrospective studies showing clear benefits. The duration of therapy should be considered to be 5 years. Gonadal ablation is an effective therapeutic intervention in metastatic male breast, and with the advent of GnRHa can easily be achieved without need for surgery. AIs may be considered in tamoxifen refractory disease, but few data are available with regard to their use in male breast cancer. There are concerns about the efficacy of oestrogen suppression with AIs given they are not able to inhibit the testicular production of oestrogen (responsible for 20% of the circulating oestrogen) and can lead to an increase in testosterone (precursor for oestrogen). Given these concerns, use of GnRHa with AI is reasonable.

Combination of endocrine and targeted therapy

In patients with HER-2 positive breast cancer, endocrine therapy can be utilised concurrently with HER-2-directed therapy in the form of trastuzumab (Herceptin) or lapatanib (Tyverb).

In HER-2-negative advanced breast cancer, the addition of the mTOR inhibitor everolimus (Afinitor) (refer to chapter 8) to exemestane (steriodial AI) results in longer disease control and is now standard of care in women who develop recurrence or progression following a non-steroidal AI.

Side effects of endocrine therapy

The most common side effects of tamoxifen are hot flushes, vaginal dryness, loss of libido and weight gain. While tamoxfen has an antagonistic effect with regard to breast cancer, its agonistic effect on the uterus and the clotting pathway can lead to its most serious adverse effects: endometrial cancer and thromboembolic disease. The benefits outweigh the risks of these rare serious adverse effects, however. A past history of endometrial cancer or thromboembolic disease precludes the use of tamoxifen, and any abnormal bleeding in women taking tamoxifen must be investigated promptly by a gynaecologist, as must any history suggestive of thromboembolic disease. Given thromboembolic issues, consideration should also be given to brief discontinuations of tamoxifen prior to any operative procedure or prolonged period of immobilisation. In premenopausal women, tamoxifen can lead to a reduction in bone density (the converse occurs in postmenopausal women) and assessment of bone health is important, particularly as such women may also have received chemotherapy, which likewise leads to a loss of bone mineral density. With AIs, the common side effects are arthralgia, myalgia, loss of libido and a reduction in bone mineral density and a resulting increase in fractures, although they are free from endometrial or thromboembolic risk. Given the associated issues with bone health, assessment for other risk factors for accelerated bone loss should be performed, vitamin D levels should be assessed and dual-energy x-ray absorptiometry (DXA) should be carried out. Vitamin D and calcium supplements or bisphosphonates can minimise the impact of AIs on bone health. Bone density

Table 9.2   Common side effects of endocrine therapy and possible interventions.

Side effect	Agent	Interventions
Hot flushes	Tamoxifen GnRHa AIs	*Nonpharmacological* • Evening dosing • Hypnotherapy • Acupuncture • Yoga *Pharmacological* • Venflaxine • Gabapentin • clonidine • Megesterol acetate Cyproterone 50 mg daily (prostate cancer only)
Vaginal dryness	Tamoxifen GnRHa AIs	Nonhormonal vaginal lubricants (such as Replens MD)
Bone health	AIs Tamoxifen (pre-menopausal) GnRHa	Modification of any pre-existing risk factors (if possible) Vitamin D and calcium bisphosphonate
Arthralgia	AIs GnRHa (prostate)	*Nonpharmacological* • Weight loss • Exercise • Physiotherapy *Pharmacological* • Analesigics • Switch to alternative AI

should be monitored regularly during treatment (see chapter 17). Similar issues regarding bone health pertain to men and women treated with GnRHa. The nongynaecological issues with tamoxfien seen in women are also observed in men. Table 9.2 summaries possible interventions for specific side effects.

Prostate cancer

Drugs targeting testosterone synthesis and signalling

The majority of circulating testosterone is produced by the Leydig cells of the adult testes in response to LH from the anterior pituitary gland, which in turn is stimulated by GnRH from the hypothalamus (Figure 9.3). Drugs that interrupt this pathway are used in the management of prostate cancer.

GnRH analogues (goserelin, leuprolin) disrupt the normal feedback loops that govern LH release and after an initial transient rise (or 'flare') result in prolonged suppression of testosterone synthesis. The flare can initially stimulate the tumour, which can result in urinary obstruction or even cord compression; therefore, a testosterone antagonist is mandatory for 2 weeks prior to administering GnRH analogues. Administered as a monthly or 3-monthly depot deep subcutaneous injection, they provide the backbone of androgen suppression and are an alternative to surgical castration for long-term use. Recently, GnRH antagonists (degaralix) have been developed which result in quicker suppression of testosterone levels without the propensity to cause flare. Nonsteroidal (cyproterone acetate) and steroidal (bicalutamide) testosterone antagonists that block binding to the androgen receptor are widely

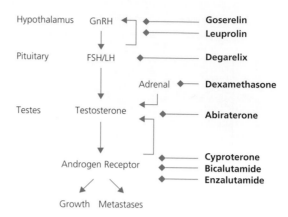

Figure 9.3 Schematic representation of the male hypothalamo-pituitary-gonadal axis, with drugs annotated.

used. Cyproterone is used as a short-term cover to prevent tumour stimulation from the flare seen at the initiation of GnRH analogues. It can also be used at a lower dose (50 mg daily) as a treatment for hot flushes associated with ADT. Bicalutamide is used in combination with LHRH antagonist for the long-term management of recurrent/metastatic disease, although the phenomenon of anti-androgen withdrawal responses (when the prostate-specific antigen (PSA) falls and the tumour responds to the stopping of bicalutamide) suggests that under certain circumstances bicalutamide may act as an agonist. A new generation of highly active testosterone antagonists (e.g. enzalutamide) is currently in development in clinical trials.

Even in the absence of testicular androgens, prostate cancer cells remain sensitive to adrenally produced testosterone. Low-dose dexamethasone (0.5 mg daily) will prevent endogenous steroid production via negative feedback inhibition of adreno-corticotropic hormone (ACTH) and the adrenal production of testosterone. The steroid may therefore be used in the treatment of advanced/metastatic disease. The antifungal ketaconzole is a nonselective inhibitior of the steroidogenic pathway and can also be used to reduce adrenal androgen production. Its broad-spectrum inhibitory effects upon the steroid synthesis pathway necessitate the concomitant use of steroids to prevent adrenal insufficiency. Abiraterone acetate is a more selective inhibitor of adrenal hormone production, through blocking of cytochrome P450(17)alpha (CYP17), but given it can result in mineralocorticoid excess (hypertension and hypokalaemia), prednisolone is coadministered. Abiraterone is licensed in prostate cancer for the treatment of metastatic castrate resistant prostate cancer.

Indications for endocrine treatment in prostate cancer

The cellular effects of androgen deprivation and radiotherapy are synergistic and a period of ADT before and during radiotherapy improves outcomes in all but the earliest tumours. This typically takes the form of monthly GnRH analogue injections (three or four prior to radiotherapy, stopped once radiotherapy is completed), although bicalutamide monotherapy is an alternative. There is no evidence of benefit in the addition of ADT to early tumours treated with brachytherapy or radical surgery (prostatectomy).

High-risk localised disease (T3/4 tumours, Gleason grades 8 and above, presenting PSA > 20 but no evidence of lymph node or bone metastases) is treated with a combination of external-beam radiotherapy and prolonged (2–3 years) adjuvant androgen deprivation. Randomised trials over the last decade have confirmed the benefit of adding ADT to radiotherapy and vice versa, with around a 10% improvement in overall survival from combination (as compared with either radiotherapy or ADT alone) at 5–10 years.

In recurrence (where PSA-detected relapse can predate symptomatic metastatic disease by months or years) or on presentation with metastatic disease, ADT forms the mainstay of treatment, in the form of either bilateral orchidectomy or long-term GnRH analogues (with 3-monthly depot injections). In well-controlled disease, an intermittent strategy of GnRH analogues (allowing the PSA to rise to a predetermined level before reinstituting treatment) has been shown to be as effective as permanent testosterone suppression and to have the potential to avoid some of the side effects (Table 9.2). However, more aggressive disease typically progresses on testosterone suppression alone after 18 months to 2 years. The therapeutic pathway then comprises maximal androgen blockade (the addition of bicalutamide) followed by withdrawal (looking for an anti-androgen withdrawal response) at each progression, usually indicated by PSA rise. Subsequent lines of treatment include daily 0.5 mg dexamethasone (response rate around 40%) followed by possible palliative chemotherapy with docetaxel for symptomatic metastatic disease. Following first-line chemotherapy, abiraterone or further chemotherapy can be considered.

Toxicity of endocrine therapy

GnRH analogues cause hot flushes, impotence and a tendency to weight gain. Longer use of bicalutamide can cause gynaecomastia, and both bicalutamide and particularly cyproterone are associated with derangement of liver function tests. Long-term androgen deprivation is a risk factor for the development of osteopenia and clinically significant osteoporosis. Identification of high-risk patients should lead to the protective use of bisphosphonates. A diagnosis of prostate cancer in itself is associated with an increased risk of cardiovascular disease, and this risk is increased further with androgen deprivation. In addition, long-term endocrine therapy in prostate cancer is associated with an increased risk of venous (but not arterial) thromboembolism.

Further reading

Bordeleau, L., Pritchard, K., Goodwin, P. & Loprinzi, C. (2007) Therapeutic options for the management of hot flashes in breast cancer survivors: an evidence-based review. *Clinical Therapeutics*, **29**, 230–241.

Davies, C., Pan, H., Godwin, J., Gray, R., Arriagada, R., Raina, V. *et al.* (2012) Long-term effects of continuing adjuvant tamoxifen to 10 years versus stopping at 5 years after diagnosis of oestrogen receptor-positive breast cancer: ATLAS, a randomised trial. *Lancet*. **381(9869)**, 805–816.

Dent, S.F., Gaspo, R., Kissner, M. & Pritchard, K.I. (2011) Aromatase inhibitor therapy: toxicities and management strategies in the treatment of postmenopausal women with hormone-sensitive early breast cancer. *Breast Cancer Research and Treatment*, **126**, 295–310.

Dowsett, M., Cuzick, J., Ingle, J., Coates, A., Forbes, J., Bliss, J. *et al.* (2010) Meta-analysis of breast cancer outcomes in adjuvant trials of aromatase inhibitors versus tamoxifen. *Journal of Clinical Oncology*, **28**, 509–518.

Early Breast Cancer Overview Group (2007) Use of luteinising-hormone-releasing hormone agonists as adjuvant treatment in premenopausal patients with hormone receptor-positive breast cancer: a meta-analysis of individual patient data from randomised adjuvant trials LHRH-agonists. *Lancet*, **369**, 1711–1723.

Early Breast Cancer Trialists' Collaborative Group (1998) Tamoxifen for early breast cancer: an overview of the randomised trials. *Lancet*, **351**, 1451–1467.

Early Breast Cancer Trialists' Collaborative Group (2011) Relevance of breast cancer hormone receptors and other factors to the efficacy of adjuvant tamoxifen: patient-level meta-analysis of randomised trials. *Lancet*, **378(9793)**, 771–781.

Korde, L.A., Zujewski, J.A., Kamin, L., Giordano, S., Domchek, S., Anderson, W.F. *et al.* (2010) Multidisciplinary meeting on male breast cancer: summary and research recommendations. *Journal of Clinical Oncology*, **28**, 2114–2122.

National Institute for Health and Clinical Excellence (2006) NICE guidance on hormonal therapies for the adjuvant treatment of early oestrogen-receptor-positive breast cancer, available from http://www.nice.org.uk (last accessed 8 March 2013).

Reid, D.M., Doughty, J., Eastell, R., Heys, S.D., Howell, A., McCloskey, E.V. *et al.* (2008) Guidance for the management of breast cancer treatment-induced bone loss: a consensus position statement from a UK Expert Group. *Cancer Treatment Reviews*, **34**, S1–S18.

Saad, F., Adachi, J.D., Brown, J.P., Canning, L.A., Gelmon, K.A., Josse, R.G. & Pritchard, K.I. (2008) Cancer treatment-induced bone loss in breast and prostate cancer. *Journal of Clinical Oncology*, **26(33)**, 5465–5476.

Van Hemelrijck, M., Garmo, H., Holmberg, L., Ingelsson, E., Bratt, O., Bill-Axelson, A. *et al.* (2010) Absolute and relative risk of cardiovascular disease in men with prostate cancer: results from the population-based PCBaSe Sweden. *Journal of Clinical Oncology*, **28(21)**, 3448–3456.

Van Hemelrijck, M., Adolfsson, J., Garmo, H., Bill-Axelson, A., Bratt, O., Ingelsson, E. *et al.* (2010) Risk of thromboembolic diseases in men with prostate cancer: results from the population-based PCBaSe Sweden. *Lancet Oncology*, **11(5)**, 450–458.

Warde, P., Mason, M., Ding, K., Kirkbride, P., Brundage, M., Cowan, R. *et al.*; NCIC CTG PR.3/MRC UK PR07 Investigators (2011) Combined androgen deprivation therapy and radiation therapy for locally advanced prostate cancer: a randomised, phase 3 trial. *Lancet*, **378(9809)**, 2104–2111.

Yap, T.A., Zivi, A., Omlin, A., de Bono, J.S. (2011) The changing therapeutic landscape of castration-resistant prostate cancer. *National Review of Clinical Oncology*, **8(10)**, 597–610.

CHAPTER 10

Biological and Targeted Therapies

Ruth E. Board[1], Jennifer W. Pang[2], Carlo Palmieri[3], and Suzy Cleator[4]

[1]Rosemere Cancer Centre, Royal Preston Hospital, Preston, UK
[2]Imperial College Healthcare NHS Trust, London, UK
[3]University of Liverpool, Department of Molecular and Clinical Cancer Medicine, The Royal Liverpool University Hospital & The Clatterbridge Cancer Centre, Liverpool, UK
[4]Imperial College Healthcare NHS Trust, London, UK

OVERVIEW

- Cancer is defined by a number of hallmarks, including the ability to divide limitlessly, evasion of cell death, the ability to develop a new blood supply and invasion and formation of metastasis
- Biological and targeted agents are treatments that aim to target these processes
- Such agents comprise monoclonal antibody treatment, tyrosine kinase inhibitors and immune modulators
- Unlike chemotherapy, these agents do not cause DNA damage directly, and their side-effect profile generally differs from those classically seen with chemotherapy
- Such agents are often used in combination with other cancer therapies, such as endocrine treatment and chemotherapy

---

Introduction

Improved scientific understanding of cancer cell biology has allowed the identification of key 'hallmarks of cancer', which include limitless ability to divide, insensitivity to growth-inhibition signals, the ability to develop blood supply (so-called 'angiogenesis'), avoidance of immune destruction and the invasion and formation of metastasis (Figure 10.1). Biological and targeted therapy encompasses a number of agents which target these critical and cancer-specific molecular pathways or processes. These agents are broadly divided into antibodies and tyrosine kinase inhibitors (TKIs; so-called 'small molecules'), and are often called 'targeted agents' or 'designer drugs'. The development of such agents is based on basic research which identifies targets within cancer cells that are critical for growth and survival. Once such discoveries have been validated as being important in human cancer, computational chemistry can be undertaken on drug libraries to identify potential candidate agents which block or modulate the target, a process often called 'rational drug design'. The whole process of taking a scientific discovery and turning it into a treatment is referred to as going 'from bench to bedside'.

ABC of Cancer Care, First Edition.
Edited by Carlo Palmieri, Esther Bird and Richard Simcock.
© 2013 John Wiley & Sons, Ltd. Published 2013 by John Wiley & Sons, Ltd.

Types of biological therapy

Tyrosine kinase inhibitors

Tyrosine kinases are cellular enzymes that are responsible for the phosphorylation of cellular proteins, leading to the activation of signal transduction cascades. Overactivity or aberrant functioning of certain tyrosine kinases has been identified as an important driver of cancer cell proliferation. TKIs are small molecules which block the function of tyrosine kinases and are thus effective as cancer therapy. Different tyrosine kinases are important in the growth of different cancers, so any TKI will only be effective in certain diseases. Imatinib mesylate (Gleevec) targets the abnormal BCR-ABL fusion protein present in over 90% of chronic myeloid leukaemia cells. Treatment of patients with imatinib in the chronic phase of chronic myeloid leukaemia (CML) leads to an over 90% response rate and significantly improved survival. The development of imatinib has been followed by a significant increase in the development of other TKIs for the treatment of cancer. The success of a TKI is often dependent on the presence or overexpression of its target protein or the presence (or absence) of a mutation within the gene coding for that particular protein. Immunohistochemistry or molecular testing of the tumour tissue may therefore be required to identify patients most likely to benefit from these drugs (e.g. the overexpression of HER-2 in breast cancer for the use of lapatinib (Tyverb) or presence of a V600E mutation (substitution of glutamic acid for valine at codon 600) in BRAF in melanoma for the use of vemurafenib (Zelboraf)) (see Chapter 11).

Unfortunately, resistance to TKIs is observed with ongoing treatment. This is often due to the acquisition of further mutations in the target protein; alternatively, it can be due to upregulation of other signalling pathways within the cell (if one pathway is blocked, the cell finds another path). In some cases, further drugs have been developed against the resistant protein, and ongoing research aims to identify mechanisms of resistance to TKIs, which could ultimately lead to the identification of other novel proteins suitable for targeting as cancer therapy. A large number of TKIs have now been developed and are in routine clinical use. These drugs are administered orally and can be given both as single agents and in combination with other systemic therapies, such as chemotherapy and endocrine therapy (see Table 10.1).

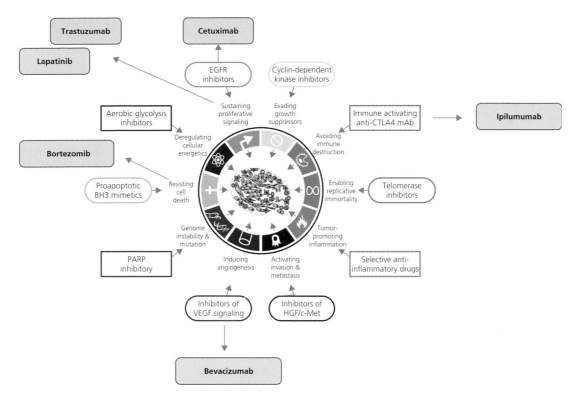

Figure 10.1 The hallmarks of cancer, with examples of licensed targeted agents. Adapted from Cell, 144 (5), Hanahan D and Weinberg RA, Hallmarks of Cancer: The Next Generation, 646–74, Copyright 2011, with permission from Elsevier.

Table 10.1 TKIs currently licensed for the treatment of cancer.

Drug name	Molecular target	Indication
Imatinib	BCR-ABL, c-kit	CML, GIST
Nilotinib	BCR-ABL	CML
Dasatanib	BCR-ABL	CML, Philadelphia positive AML & ALL
Erlotinib	EGFR	NSCLC
Gefitinib	EGFR	NSCLC with EGFR mutations
Crizotinib	ALK, c-MET	NSCLC with ELM4-ALK fusion protein
Lapatinib	EGFR, HER-2	HER-2 overexpressing breast cancer
Sunitinib	VEGFR, PDGFR, c-kit	Renal cell cancer, GIST, pancreatic neuroendocrine tumours
Sorafenib	VEGFR, RAF, c-kit	Renal cell cancer, hepatocellular cancer
Vemurafenib	BRAF	Metastatic melanoma with BRAF mutations
Temsirolimus	mTOR	Renal cell cancer
Everolimus	mTOR	Renal cell cancer, breast cancer
Bortezomib	Proteasome inhibitor	Multiple myeloma

EGFR, epidermal growth factor receptor; VEGFR, vascular endothelial growth factor receptor; PDGFR, platelet-derived growth factor receptor; CML, chronic myeloid leukaemia; AML, acute myeloid leukaemia; ALL, acute lymphoblastic leukaemia; GIST, gastrointestinal stromal tumour; NSCLC, non-small-cell lung cancer.

Monoclonal antibodies

Monoclonal antibodies (mABs) can be divided into chimeric (imab) and humanised (umab) forms (Figure 10.2), and have an established role in the treatment of cancer. A number have been approved for clinical use (Table 10.2). Classically, tumour-directed mABs bind to a surface molecule that is driving proliferation of malignant cells, such as members of the epidermal growth factor receptor (EGFR) family HER-1 and HER-2. This is illustrated by the mAB trastuzumab (Herceptin), which targets surface HER-2, a cell-surface receptor that is overexpressed and therefore a potential 'driver' in 10–15% of breast cancers. By binding to the surface component of HER-2, trastuzumab suppresses HER-2 signalling

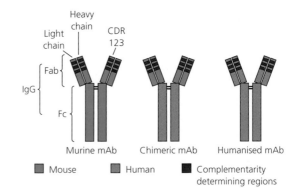

Figure 10.2 Structure of monoclonal antibodies: chimeric versus humanised. Reprinted from The Lancet, 355 (9205), Breedveld FC, Therapeutic monoclonal antibodies, 735–40, Copyright (2010), with permission from Elsevier.

Table 10.2 Monoclonal antibodies currently licensed for the treatment of cancer.

Drug name	Molecular target	Indication
bevacizumab	VEGF	In combination with chemotherapy for breast and ovarian cancer, CRC and NSCLC In combination with interferon alfa-2a for renal cell carcinoma
cetuximab	EGFR	In combination with radiotherapy or chemotherapy for SCC of head and neck CRC (KRAS nonmutated)
panitumumab	EGFR	CRC (KRAS nonmutated)
traztuzumab	HER-2	HER-2-positive breast cancer HER-2-positive gastric cancer
rituximab	CD20	With chemotherapy for treatment of symptomatic stage III and IV follicular lymphoma Monotherapy as maintenance therapy in stage III and IV follicular lymphoma in chemotherapy-induced remission In combination with chemotherapy for CLL In combination with chemotherapy for CD20-positive diffuse large-B-cell lymphoma
90Y-Ibritumomab tiuxetan (Zevalin)	CD20	Rituximab relapsed or refractory CD20-positive follicular B-cell NHL First-line consolidation therapy after remission induction in previously untreated patients with follicular lymphoma
alemtuzumab	CD52	CLL
ofatumumab	CD20	CLL
ipilimumab	CTLA4	Metastatic melanoma

VEGF, vascular endothelial growth factor; CRC, colorectal cancer; NSCLC, non-small-cell lung cancer; EGFR, epidermal growth factor receptor; SCC, squamous cell carcinoma; CLL, chronic lymphocytic leukaemia.

and triggers immune-mediated cell kill (antibody-dependent cell-mediated cytotoxicity, ADCC). Trastuzumab (Herceptin) is associated with improved survival in the setting of HER-2 over-expressing early and secondary breast cancer, whereas no activity has been reliably demonstrated in breast cancers without HER-2 over-expression. Pertuzumab (Perjeta) blocks the dimerisation of HER-2 with its family member HER-3, and in advanced breast cancer when combined with trastuzumab results in improved survival compared to trastuzumab alone.

Cetuximab (Erbitux) and panitumumab (Vectibix), which bind to surface EGFR (otherwise known as HER-1), have proven activity in KRAS wild-type colorectal cancer. Mutations in the KRAS gene, which is downstream of EGFR, can drive colorectal cancer growth independent of EGFR signaling; therefore, blocking upstream EGFR is only effective in cases where KRAS mutation is absent. In order to grow and metastasise, many cancers rely on the parallel development of tumour vasculature. This process, known as angiogenesis, is driven by a number of local growth factors, including vascular endothelial growth factor (VEGF). Bevacizumab

(Avastin), a mAB that binds VEGF, inhibits angiogenesis and may normalise tumour vasculature to aid in delivery of other anticancer agents. Bevacizumab in combination with chemotherapy has been shown to be effective in a number of cancer types, including colorectal and renal cell cancer.

More recently, the mAB ipilimumab has been shown to improve survival in advanced melanoma. Ipilimumab targets cytotoxic T-lymphocyte associated antigen 4 (CTLA4) expressed on T-cells. By neutralising CTLA4, ipilimumab (Yervoy) prevents downregulation of T-cells, leading to a sustained immune response and recognition and destruction of 'foreign' melanoma cells.

mABs and delivery of chemotherapy or radiotherapy

An attraction of mABs as therapeutic agents is the fact that other cytotoxic therapies can be bound to the antibody, directing the cytotoxic straight to the disease. For example, 90Y-ibritumomab tiuxetan (Zevalin) consists of an anti-CD20 mAB linked to yttrium-90 (90Y). This facilitates delivery of cytotoxic doses of short-acting radiation to the CD20-positive cells in B-cell non-Hodgkin lymphoma. Trastuzumab emtansine (TDM-1 / Kadcyla) consists of the anti-HER-2 antibody trastuzumab conjugated to the potent antimicrotubule agent DM1 (a maytansine derivative), and this delivers chemotherapy to HER-2-positive breast cancer cells.

Targeted therapies that regulate events in the nucleus

Most targeted therapies used in cancer target processes outside the nucleus. However, some influence the processes of gene transcription within the nucleus (Table 10.3). These include vorinostat (Zolinza), which inhibits the activity of a group of enzymes called histone deacetylases (HDACs). HDACs remove chemical groups called acetyl groups from many different proteins, including those involved in regulating gene expression. Another class, the retinoids, are chemically related to vitamin A and bind to and activate nuclear receptors known as retinoic acid and retinoid X receptors. Once activated, these receptors regulate the expression of genes that control processes such as cell growth and differentiation. Figure 10.3 gives examples of targeted agents and where they act.

Interferon and interleukin

Interferon and interleukin are naturally occurring cytokines that are used to stimulate the immune system against cancer cells. Their use in cancer either as single agents or in combination with chemotherapy is limited to a small number of tumour types. Two

Table 10.3 Targeted therapies that regulate gene expression.

Drug name	Molecular target	Indication
Vorinostat Romidepsin	Histone deacetylase inhibitors	Cutaneous T-cell lymphoma
Bexarotene	Retinoid X receptors	Cutaneous T-cell lymphoma
Alitretinoin	Retinoic acid receptors and retinoid X receptors	AIDS-related Kaposi sarcoma
Tretinoin	Retinoic acid receptors	Acute promyelocytic leukemia

agents that are currently in used are interleukin-2 (Aldesleukin) and interferon alpha (Roferon, Intron A), which are used in renal cell cancer, malignant melanoma, multiple myeloma and hairy-cell leukaemia. High-dose interleukin-2 has been shown to achieve long-term remission in a small number of highly selected renal cell cancer patients.

The side effects can be significant depending on the doses administered and include flu-like symptoms, fatigue, hypotension, nausea, drops in blood count and mental disturbance. The use of these drugs has diminished since the introduction of a number of targeted agents.

Vaccines

Vaccines are developed against cancer-specific antigens with the aim of stimulating the patient's immune system to recognise and attack the cancer cells. To date, only one has been approved for use. This is called sipuleucel-T (Provenge) and is indicated for men with metastatic prostate cancer that is refractory to endocrine therapy. It is designed to stimulate an immune response to prostatic acid phosphatase (PAP), an antigen found on prostate cancer cells. Sipuleucel-T requires the extraction and stimulation in a laboratory of the patient's own antigen-presenting cells (APCs) with a fusion protein consisting of PAP fused to granulocyte–macrophage colony-stimulating factor, an immune-cell activator which enhances antigen presentation. These cells are then infused back, causing activation of the T-cells within the immune system, which then kill the cancer cells.

Development of cancer vaccines remains a challenging area for cancer treatment, but vaccines which reduce the incidence of cancer are in routine clinical use, including ones against the human

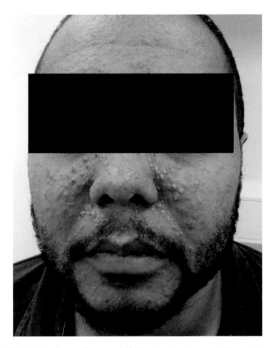

Figure 10.4 Typical acneiform rash following treatment with cetuximab, a monoclonal antibody against EGFR used in the treatment of colorectal cancer.

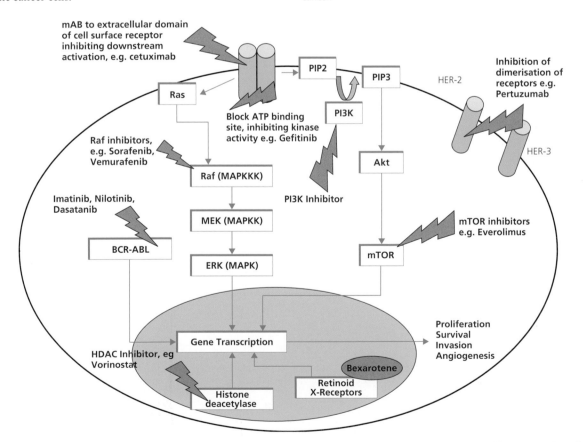

Figure 10.3 Examples of transmembrane receptors, intracellular pathways and factors involved in nuclear transcription targeted by mABs and small molecules.

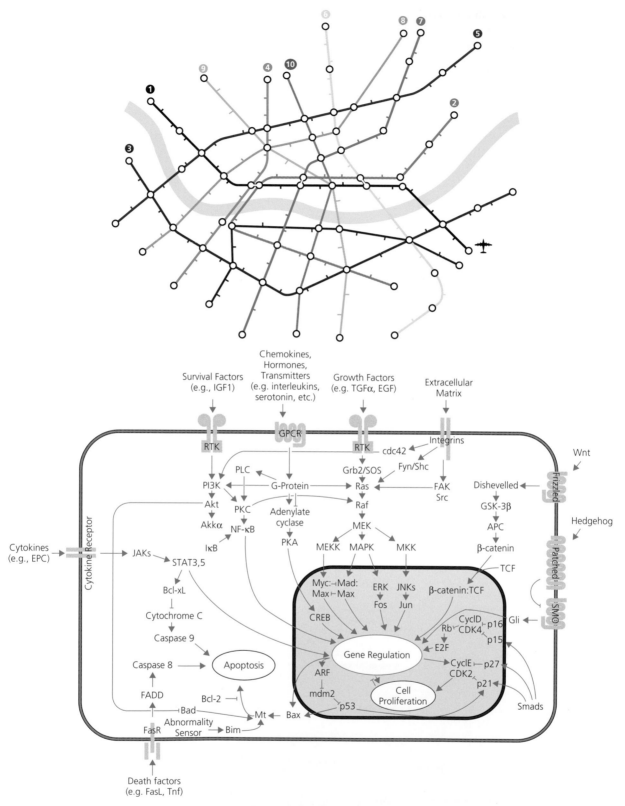

Figure 10.5 Pictorial explanation of resistance to targeted therapies in cancer cells. Adapted from Cell, 100 (1), Hanahan D and Weinberg RA, Hallmarks of Cancer, 57–70, Copyright (2000), with permission from Elsevier. Generic underground map, modified with permission from iStockphoto.com.

papilloma virus (HPV) (Gardasil and Cervarix), which can lead to cervical cancer and hepatitis B, which can lead to hepatocellular carcinoma.

Colony stimulating factors

Colony stimulating factors (CSFs), or haematopoietic growth factors, are biological agents that are used in supportive therapy rather than as direct cancer treatments. They encourage stem cells in the bone marrow to produce white cells and red cells. Granulocyte colony stimulating factors (GCSFs) are used increase the number of white blood cells, while erythropoietin increases the number of red blood cells.

Toxicities

Due to their novel mechanism of action, TKIs and mABs have very different toxicities from traditional chemotherapy. Given their structure, there is a risk of allergic reactions with infusion of mABs. The most common toxicities of these drugs include diarrhoea and skin rashes. Often the toxicity relates to the mechanism of action of the drug (e.g. drugs targeting angiogenesis lead to an increased bleeding tendency), but in many cases the mechanism behind the toxicity is unclear and can be unusual and unexpected. For example, trastuzumab was identified as causing a measurable decrease in left ventricular function and symptomatic heart failure in a small proportion of patients, and cardiac monitoring in treated patients is now routine. This is due to interference with HER-2 signalling in myocytes. If it occurs, it is generally considered reversible. The agent vemurafenib in melanoma is known to give rise to squamous cell skin cancers in some patients, due to a paradoxical activation of the cell signalling system.

There is some evidence to suggest that the development of a rash after treatment with an EGFR inhibitor (see Figure 10.4) or the development of hypertension with therapies targeting VEGR may identify a group of patients with a higher response rate, but this is a controversial area and research is ongoing to identify biomarkers of response to these novel agents.

Treatment of side effects is generally symptomatic but may require dose reduction. While they are traditionally considered safer than chemotherapy, it is important to recognise that the side effects of biological agents can be significant, and there is a risk of life-threatening toxicities with these therapies. In particular, patients on oral targeted therapies need counselling regarding potential toxicities and should be told to stop and seek medical attention if they occur.

The future

Advances in our understanding and knowledge of cancer biology, driven by coordinated scientific projects like the Genome Project and ENCODE, among other things, are leading to a rapid expansion in possible targets. This in turn will lead to new drugs entering clinical trials and becoming licensed. It is critical that as part of the development of these agents in clinical trials, markers predictive of benefit (biomarkers) are identified to limit futile drug exposure, with all its inherent risks of toxicity, as well as to ensure that resources are not wasted, given the inherently high cost of such new agents (see Chapter 11). The cost of these agents also means that society faces difficult decisions regarding how to fund these drugs and how to weigh the benefit of a drug which may only extend life by a few months in the first instance against its cost. Already access to some of these new agents is often restricted on health economy grounds.

Upfront or acquired resistance is a major limiting factor to targeted agents. This can arise from pathway redundancy: many cancers are not purely dependent on one sole driver (so-called 'oncogene addiction') and cancer cells can develop further mutations as a result of their inherent genomic instability, which enables them to circumvent the inhibitory effects of the targeted agents (Figure 10.5). Understanding and modulating these resistance mechanisms is key if more successful agents are to be developed.

Further reading

Breedveld, F.C. (2010) Therapeutic monoclonal antibodies. *Lancet*, **355(9205)**, 735–740.

Giaccone, G. & Soria, J.-C. (2007) *Targeted Therapies in Oncology*. CRC Press, Boca Raton.

Hanahan, D. & Weinberg, R.A. (2000) Hallmarks of cancer. *Cell*, **100(1)**, 57–70.

Hanahan, D. & Weinberg, R. (2011) Hallmarks of cancer: the next generation. *Cell*, **144**, 646–674.

Kerbel, R. (2008) Tumor angiogenesis. *New England Journal of Medicine*, **358**, 2039–2049.

Laurent-Puig, P., Lievre, A. & Blons, H. (2009) Mutations and response to epidermal growth factor receptor inhibitors. *Clinical Cancer Research*, **15(4)**, 1133–1139.

National Institute for Health and Clinical Excellence cancer guidance topics, http://guidance.nice.org.uk/Topic/Cancer (last accessed 8 March 2013).

CHAPTER 11

Trials in Cancer Care

Evandro de Azambuja[1], David Cameron[2], and Janet E. Brown[3]

[1]BrEAST Data Centre, Jules Bordet Institute, Brussels, Belgium
[2]University of Edinburgh, Edinburgh, UK
[3]University of Leeds, St James's University Hospital, Leeds, UK

OVERVIEW

- Clinical trials in cancer are highly regulated patient studies usually designed to determine the safety and efficacy of new treatments
- They are fundamentally designed to test scientific hypotheses, and require attention to detail in both design and statistical analysis
- Phase I trials are primarily concerned with safety and toxicity and seek to establish the maximum safe dose for a new drug
- Phase II trials extend safety data, but are concerned with efficacy and establishing dose
- Phase III trials assess whether the novel treatment or agent is better than the best current standard of care
- All clinical trials must be carried out in strict accordance with pre-agreed ethical procedures and are designed such that risks are minimised. For trials involving drugs, there are regulatory requirements around the reporting of side effects to help ensure patient safety

Introduction

Biomarkers are increasingly used in trials and in clinical practice. These are readily measured biological parameters which can predict whether a patient will respond to a particular treatment and which therefore permit tailored treatment.

What are clinical trials?

Clinical trials are vital in the development of cancer therapies. Each attempts to answer specific questions around prevention, screening, diagnosis and treatment. Clinical trials may compare a new treatment (experimental) with an available one (comparator or standard). They have a protocol, in which the objectives, patient group, end point and type of analysis are clearly specified prior to beginning. Key to the success of clinical trials are patient participation and altruism.

Clinical trials can be observational or interventional. In the former, individuals are observed over time and the outcomes are measured (e.g. lifestyle and the development of cancer). In the latter, research subjects are given an intervention and health changes are measured.

Box 11.1 list the different categories of trial, according to the US National Institutes of Health (NIH).

Box 11.1 Five categories of clinical trial

1 Treatment trials: test experimental, new drugs.
2 Prevention trials: evaluate how to prevent a certain disease or to avoid relapses.
3 Diagnostic trials: try to find better tests or procedures for a certain disease.
4 Screening trials: test the best way to detect certain diseases.
5 Quality of life trials: explore ways of improving the subject's comfort.

The 'road map' for taking an idea into routine clinical practice is well defined for drugs; this chapter will therefore largely focus on this group of trials. Similar concepts apply to other treatments, such as surgery and radiotherapy, although the regulatory framework is less precise and the distinction between phase I and phase II studies is often blurred.

The drug development process

Historically there were large elements of chance in the discovery of new drugs. Drug discovery now depends on an understanding of the underlying molecular pathways of a specific cancer. Many of the initial discoveries, which subsequently yield molecular targets and then novel drugs, are derived from basic laboratory research. Any novel agent needs to go through a rigorous series of *in vitro* tests to demonstrate its potential for efficacy and specificity before it progresses into a preclinical stage. Preclinical tests include animal testing for further characterisation, including such factors as best route of administration, pharmacokinetics (metabolism and elimination of drugs) and both safety and efficacy, before the drug can be considered for human use.

Only a small minority of agents tested reach clinical trial. A drug may take 6 years to pass all preclinical tests. The subsequent

ABC of Cancer Care, First Edition.
Edited by Carlo Palmieri, Esther Bird and Richard Simcock.
© 2013 John Wiley & Sons, Ltd. Published 2013 by John Wiley & Sons, Ltd.

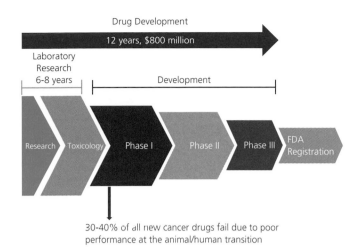

30-40% of all new cancer drugs fail due to poor performance at the animal/human transition

Figure 11.1 Drug development is an expensive, slow, long and risky business. Several drugs tested in the laboratory do not pass this step and many of those that do pass it will fail due to poor performance at the animal/human transition. Very few drugs will get US Food and Drug Administration (FDA) approval after almost 12 years of testing.

time required for clinical development and approval from regulatory agencies is typically around 8 years (Figure 11.1) – a long interval between concept and patient use. The process is expensive and the attrition rate is high, since many potential drugs fail to meet the stringent regulatory requirements, even at the final stages.

Phases of clinical trials

Trials testing new treatments are normally divided into four phases (I, II, III and IV), each of which has a specific research aim (see Table 11.1).

Table 11.1 Summary of different phases of clinical trials.

Clinical trial phase	Tumour types	Number of patients	Main objectives
I	Various	Tens	To find a safe dose To decide how the new treatment should be given To see how the new treatment affects the human body
II	Selected	Tens–hundreds	To determine whether the new treatment has an effect on a certain cancer To see how the new treatment affects the human body
III	Selected	Hundreds–thousands	To compare the new treatment (or new use of a treatment) with the current standard treatment
IV	Selected	Variable	To further assess the long-term safety and effectiveness of a new treatment

Phase I

Phase I trials are the first stage of testing of a new drug in human subjects. They are usually small trials (maximum of 50 patients) and are designed to assess the safety, pharmacodynamics, pharmacokinetics and tolerability of a therapy. Normally, there is a dose escalation to identify the drug limiting toxicity (DLT) and the maximum tolerated dose (MTD), in order to define the appropriate dose and schedule for further efficacy-focussed testing in patients.

Subjects are often either cancer patients who have used all conventional therapies for their tumour type and in whom prognosis is limited or patients for whom there is no standard treatment. Since efficacy is not the main objective of phase I clinical trials, different tumour types may be included in the same trial.

Phase II

Phase II clinical trials involve larger numbers of particpants (tens to hundreds) and are designed to assess how well a therapy works in cancer patients. In this phase, trials usually focus on a particular type of cancer (e.g. breast cancer) or a particular subtype (e.g. HER-2 positive breast cancer). These trials continue to assess drug safety, with a focus on any concerns picked up in the phase I studies. Patient safety is paramount. These studies can pick up toxicity concerns that may not have been apparent in the phase I trial (e.g. cardiotoxicity with trastuzumab). Phase IIA clinical trials are designed to assess dosing requirements, whereas phase IIB clinical trials are designed to study efficacy. In some cases, phase I and phase II trials are combined, to report on both efficacy and toxicities. Normally, results are reported as overall response rate (ORR, i.e. tumour shrinkage rate), clinical benefit (combination of complete and partial responses plus stable disease), time to progression or progression-free survival (in the case of randomised studies). At this stage, these trials can be a case series (nonrandomised) or randomised clinical trials, with the latter requiring more patients in order to enable comparisons across the arms of the study.

The key focus of a phase II study should be to produce the evidence base that justifies a subsequent phase III trial – though this is not always apparent from the design of some phase II studies. It is useful when designing a phase II study to have a concept of an outline phase III design, and to understand how the phase II results will inform the decision of whether to proceed to phase III or not.

Phase III

Phase III clinical trials need to be capable of definitive comparison between interventions. They are therefore almost always controlled, multicentre and randomised, and involve large numbers of patients (hundreds to thousands). These trials are often multinational, which ensures access to a sufficiently large patient population, but also allows them to benefit from being more broadly representative of the pattern of a particular disease. There is a definitive assessment of how effective a treatment is as compared to the current 'gold standard' treatment. Some trials may contain a placebo arm in order to minimise bias, particularly in the reporting of efficacy and side effects.

Phase III trials usually aim to demonstrate a clinically relevant benefit, normally either overall survival or progression-free survival.

Sometimes the purpose may be to show that a new treatment is just as good as (non-inferior to) the current standard in terms of the primary endpoint, but is in some way better for the patient (e.g. shorter or involving less-toxic therapy).

In addition to the primary end point, there are usually a number of secondary objectives, such as different measures of outcome (e.g. distant disease-free survival). Safety and, sometimes, quality of life are reported as secondary end points.

Appropriate phase III trials are required by regulatory agencies to confirm the efficacy and acceptable toxicity of a given drug prior to registration and licensing.

Phase IV

Phase IV clinical trials are less common and occur after a drug receives approval to be marketed. These trials involve the safety surveillance of a given drug and technical support for pharmacovigilance departments. Phase IV studies may be required by regulatory agencies or may be undertaken by the sponsoring company. Objectives are to find new markets for a given drug, test drug interactions or monitor uses in specific populations. Rare and/or long-term adverse events reporting is an important phase IV objective.

Ethical principles of clinical trials

It is an international requirement that trial patients are protected from excess risk. There is a robust ethical approval framework around initiation of any protocol. Most trials involve individuals being offered an option to enrol in the research, but there are examples where individual consent is not deemed necessary by the ethics committee. In a 'cluster' randomisation, whole groups of patients are randomised in order to measure the benefit of an intervention at the population level, such as with cancer screening.

The 1964 Declaration of Helsinki set out the fundamental principles regarding the use of human subjects in medical research: respect for the individual, the right of self-determination and the right to make informed decisions regarding participation initially and during any research.

Before entering a study, patients must be given appropriate time to read and discuss the 'patient information sheet' before signing an 'informed consent form'. Investigators require approval from the local ethics authority, which ensures that the clinical trial protects its subjects' rights with respect to its conduct. Trials are overseen by an independent data monitoring committee (IDMC), which has responsibility for safeguarding the interests of trial participants. Efficacy and safety data (not available to those running the trial) are provided to the IDMC, and early study closure can be recommended if there are concerns or if the benefits in one study arm are so clear as to make continuation unethical.

Good clinical practice

Studies must be carried out according to the set of internationally recognised ethical and scientific standards called Good Clinical Practice (GCP). This lays out guidelines on the protection of subjects, study conduct and the role and responsibilities of all those involved in the study. In the European Union, this is laid out in the EU Clinical Trials Directive (2001/20/EC), and in the UK in the Medicines for Human Use (Clinical Trials) Regulations 2004.

Trial design

Careful attention is required in the design of a trial. A poorly designed trial is neither good science nor good clinical practice.

Statistical considerations are key. For a study asking a definitive question about the benefits of a new intervention, a randomised design is usually used. Randomisation minimises 'bias'; it ensures that when a comparison is made between two groups, the only key difference between the groups is the intervention itself, rather than patient or disease characteristics.

Strongly linked to the design is the 'power' of a study. This can be considered the chance of missing a real effect. If too few patients are included in a study then natural variations in outcomes (largely due to unknown or poorly understood biological characteristics of the patients and their diseases) may lead to no difference in outcome being reported. This highlights the importance of a distinction between phase II and phase III studies (even if both phases are randomised): the phase II study aims to demonstrate enough evidence of a benefit to justify the phase III, which in turn seeks to get a more precise estimate of the true effect and of whether clinical practice should change. There are examples of cancer drugs that produced impressive improvements in outcome in phase II trials but had much less convincing results in phase III, such that those drugs have not entered routine practice.

Biomarkers in cancer trials

Biomarkers are defined as 'a characteristic that is objectively measured and evaluated as an indicator of normal biological processes, or pharmacologic responses to a therapeutic intervention' (Biomarker Definitions Working Group 2001). Accordingly, a biomarker can be any molecule present within body fluids (e.g. blood, cerebrospinal fluid, urine) or a tissue-based detectable molecular characteristic. Biomarkers have three clinical utilities: (1) prognostic markers, which predict disease; (2) predictive biomarkers, which predict the degree of therapy response; and (3) surrogate end points: measured molecular alterations which predict treatment efficacy more quickly than traditional outcomes such as overall survival (see Figure 11.1). Using biomarkers as 'surrogate outcomes' can greatly accelerate the process of drug development.

Modern biomarkers can be either altered DNA sequences (discovered by genomics), altered protein levels (discovered by proteomics) or altered metabolite levels (discovered by metabolomics) (see Figure 11.2). In cancer trials, patient samples can be collected for biomarker discovery or later validation. Sample collection with linked clinical outcome data is an important resource with which to optimise future therapy and so enable post hoc biomarker discovery.

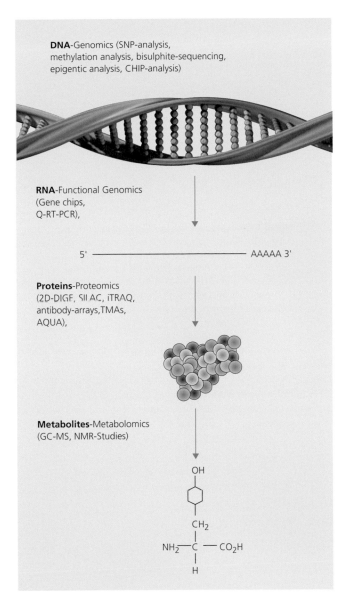

DNA-Genomics (SNP-analysis, methylation analysis, bisulphite-sequencing, epigentic analysis, CHIP-analysis)

RNA-Functional Genomics (Gene chips, Q-RT-PCR),

5' ——————————————— AAAAA 3'

Proteins-Proteomics (2D-DIGE, SILAC, iTRAQ, antibody-arrays,TMAs, AQUA),

Metabolites-Metabolomics (GC-MS, NMR-Studies)

Figure 11.2 Molecular biomarkers can be altered sequences of DNA or amplification/deletion of genes (revealed by genomics), changes in the level of gene expression revealed through measurements of mRNA (studied by functional genomics), alterations in the amount or sequence of proteins (studied by proteomics) or changes in metabolite levels (studied by metabolomics). These four methods for biomarker detection relate to the biomolecules which encode and process biological information, from genes (DNA) to mRNA to proteins and eventually to altered metabolites.

Some trials now recruit subjects based on expression of a biomarker rather than the stage of their cancer. The biomarker may suggest particular sensitivity to the test agent, or else it may itself be the target for the new drug. These trials are 'enriched' and result in a more robust test; the likelihood of a beneficial effect being missed because of population heterogeneity is thus reduced.

Biomarker discovery: a historical perspective

Historically, biomarkers have been discovered by empirical study. Prostate-specific antigen (PSA) is a clinically useful biomarker

of prostate cancer. The antibody CA125 detects a glycoprotein elevated in ovarian cancer. Low levels of serum CA125 may predict progression-free survival in patients treated with paclitaxel chemotherapy.

These biomarkers have limitations. CA125 may be elevated in benign conditions, such as cirrhosis, and PSA is elevated in benign prostatic hyperplasia and prostatitis. There are many cancers with no useful biomarkers. In view of these limitations, attempts have been made to identify panels of biomarkers and so increase specificity and sensitivity. Modern molecular biomarkers now include genes, alterations in gene expression and protein or metabolite levels (see Figure 11.3). Modern DNA sequencing technologies are quick and affordable enough to be moved from a research technique to phase III trials, and in some cases standard clinical care (see Table 11.2). They can also be used on formalin-fixed paraffin-embedded tissue samples that have been stored for long periods.

Approaches to the detection of biomarkers: genomics, proteomics, metabolomics

Genomic alterations within cancers take one of three different forms: (1) gene amplification/deletion, where a cancer-promoting or cancer-suppressing gene is either amplified by duplication or deleted by excision of a region of the chromosome; (2) single-nucleotide polymorphisms (SNPs), where a single base change within a cancer-promoting/suppressing gene alters the function of the protein encoded; and (3) altered gene transcription, where the level of expression from the gene is altered, thus altering the level of the protein encoded. These alterations may be detected by array-based technologies, and this can inform clinical decision making.

Table 11.2 Clinically relevant biomarkers in current practice and their uses.

Disease	Biomarker	Advantage
Colorectal cancer	KRAS/BRAF-activating gene mutations	Presence of mutation identifies patients with tumours less likely to respond to anti-EGFR-pathway antibody therapies (cetuximab/panitumumab)
Lung cancer	EGFR	Identifying mutations in EGFR helps predict response to anti-EGFR therapy (gefitinib)
Melanoma	BRAF	40–60% of cutaneous melanomas contain a BRAF mutation, which predicts for response to vemurafenib therapy
Breast cancer	30 or 21 gene panels	Expression of gene profiles predicts for a tumour's recurrence risk and therefore helps better estimate the absolute benefit of adjuvant chemotherapy. Commercially available tests such as the 'Oncotype' 21 gene score are increasingly used in breast cancer

EGFR, endothelial growth factor receptor.

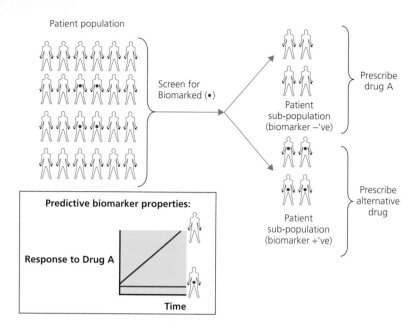

Figure 11.3 Biomarkers can be used to assess the response of patients to a drug treatment. In the example illustrated, the presence of the biomarker predicts poor response to drug A. Use of an initial screen for this biomarker thus detects the subpopulation of patients within the treatment population who will respond to treatment with drug A, and this can inform subsequent treatment decisions.

Further reading

Biomarkers Definitions Working Group (2001) Biomarkers and surrogate endpoints: preferred definitions and conceptual framework. *Clinical Pharmacology & Therapeutics*, **69(3)**, 89–95.

British Medical Journal (n.d.) Study design and choosing a statistical test, http://www.bmj.com/about-bmj/resources-readers/publications/statistics-square-one/13-study-design-and-choosing-statisti (last accessed 8 March 2013).

Keating, P. & Cambrosio, A. (2012) *Cancer on Trial: Oncology as a New Style of Practice*. University of Chicago Press, Chicago.

National Institute for Health Research Cancer Research Network Web site, www.ncrn.org.uk.

CHAPTER 12

Oncological Emergencies

Thomas E. Newsom-Davis[1] and Mohammed Rizwanullah[2]

[1]Chelsea and Westminster Healthcare NHS Foundation Trust, London, UK
[2]Beatson West of Scotland Cancer Centre, Glasgow, UK

OVERVIEW

- There are, on average, five emergency admissions of cancer patients each day per hospital in the UK
- Neutropenic sepsis is usually managed by empirical broad-spectrum antibiotics. Antibiotics should be given as soon as possible
- Metastatic spinal cord compression is challenging to diagnose early, but this is crucial for better outcome
- Superior vena cava obstruction (SVCO) is due to malignancy in 90% of cases – usually lung cancer
- Abnormalities of calcium and magnesium are common and often require intravenous management

Table 12.1 Oncology emergencies (from Appendix 3, National Cancer Action Team 2011).

Caused by the systemic treatment of cancer	Neutropenic sepsis
	Uncontrolled nausea and vomiting
	Extravasation injury
	Acute hypersensitivity/anaphylaxis
	Complication of central venous access devices
	Uncontrolled diarrhoea
	Uncontrolled mucositis
	Hypomagnasaemia
Caused by radiotherapy	Acute skin reactions
	Uncontrolled nausea and vomiting
	Uncontrolled diarrhoea
	Uncontrolled mucositis
	Radiation pneumonitis
	Acute cerebral/other CNS oedema
Caused directly by malignant disease	Pleural effusion
	Pericardial effusion
	Lymphangitis carcinomatosis
	SVCO
	Abdominal ascites
	Hypercalcaemia of malignancy
	Metastatic spinal cord compression
	Cerebral space occupying lesions

CNS, central nervous system; SVCO, superior vena cava obstruction.

Acute oncology: the management of oncology emergencies

Oncology emergencies are common. In the UK they accounted for 273 000 admissions in 2006/7, an increase of 30% over the preceding decade, meaning that a typical hospital will acutely admit an average of five oncology patients per day. Oncology emergencies (Table 12.1) may be caused by treatments for cancer (e.g. chemotherapy and radiotherapy) or can be related to the cancer diagnosis itself.

In 2008/9, recognition of the workload of patients presenting to hospital with oncology emergencies led to the development of the field of acute oncology. With combined expertise from general medicine, acute medicine and oncology, all hospitals in the UK with an emergency department are required to have an acute oncology service.

Neutropenic sepsis

Chemotherapy is widely associated with myelosupression. The neutrophil part of the white blood cell population is particularly susceptible to chemotherapy and neutropenia is therefore common. It renders the patient highly vulnerable to bacterial infection.

Febrile neutropenia (a high temperature in the presence of low neutrophil count) is the commonest cause of treatment-related hospitalisation in cancer patients and requires prompt recognition of symptoms and appropriate investigations (Table 12.2). Patients on chemotherapy should be educated to report fever immediately, and most cancer centres have protocols to ensure that patients receive antibiotics as quickly as possible. This is often audited in terms of 'door to needle' time. A prompt response is vital as, without appropriate immunity, infection can quickly develop into a neutropenic sepsis with hypotension and tachycardia. Neutropenic sepsis is not always associated with a fever, and therefore other potential hallmarks of infection (e.g. sore throat and cough) should also be referred and investigated promptly.

Mortality has steadily decreased over the past 40 years and is now 5% for solid organ tumours; however, it can be as high as 11% in some haematological malignancies.

ABC of Cancer Care, First Edition.
Edited by Carlo Palmieri, Esther Bird and Richard Simcock.
© 2013 John Wiley & Sons, Ltd. Published 2013 by John Wiley & Sons, Ltd.

Table 12.2 Neutropenic sepsis.

Definition of neutropenic sepsis	• ANC < 0.5×10^9 per litre (or expected to rapidly fall to <0.5×10^9 per litre) • Oral temperature > 38.5 °C (or two consecutive readings of >38 °C)
Initial investigations	• FBC and coagulation screen • U&E, LFT, Ca^{++}, Mg^{++}, CRP • Blood cultures (peripheral and from central line if present) • Urinalysis, microscopy and culture • Sputum microscopy and culture (if productive cough) • Stool microscopy and culture • Chest radiograph

ANC, absolute neutrophil count; FBC, full blood count; U&E, urea and electrolytes; LFT, liver function test; CRP, C-reactive protein.

Microbiology

The causative pathogens vary between geographical areas and are often difficult to identify (less than 30% of blood cultures yield clinically significant result). Historically more common, Gram-negative organisms (*E. coli*, klebsiella, enterobacter) are now seen less frequently, while Gram positives (staphylococcus, streptococcus, enterococcus) represent 70% of identified organisms. There has been a recent increase in the prevalence of antibiotic-resistant organisms such as methicillin-resistant *Staphylococcus aureus* (MRSA), vancomycin-resistant enterococci (VRE) and extended-spectrum beta-lactamase (ESBL)-producing Gram-negative bacteria.

Antimicrobial treatment

Prompt initiation of empirical broad-spectrum antimicrobials has been the cornerstone of the management of neutropenic sepsis for decades. Local guidelines will reflect local resistance patterns, but treatment usually involves a β-lactam agent that has activity against Gram-negative organisms, including *pseudomonas* (e.g. ceftazidime, piperacillin/tazobactam, meropenem). An aminoglycoside (e.g. gentamicin, amikacin) may be indicated in unstable, septic patients. The addition of glycopeptides (e.g. vancomycin, teicoplanin) should be considered in patients with known or suspected MRSA carriage.

The majority of patients with neutropenic sepsis follow an uneventful clinical course and do not require prolonged admissions for intravenous antibiotics. Various scoring systems have been developed to identify 'low-risk' individuals, the Multinational Association for Supportive Care in Cancer (MASCC) scoring index being perhaps the best known (Figure 12.1). Such patients can safely be managed with single-agent oral antibiotics (e.g. ciprofloxacin), with the aim of early discharge.

Granulocyte colony stimulating factor

Routine use of granulocyte colony stimulating factor (GCSF) is not indicated during neutropenic sepsis, and is instead reserved for medically unstable patients or those thought to be at high risk of infection complications or poor outcome. It may be used

		Yes	No	Score
Does the patient have a solid tumour or lymphoma?		4	0	
Is the patient dehydrated or requiring IV fluids?		0	3	
Is the systolic BP <90 mmHg?		0	5	
How sick is the patient now?	No or mild symptoms	5	0	
	Moderate symptoms	3	0	
	Severe symptoms	0	0	
Is the patient <60 years old?		2	0	
Does the patient have COPD?		0	4	
Did the patient develop febrile neutropenia while an inpatient?		0	3	
Total MASCC score				

(a)

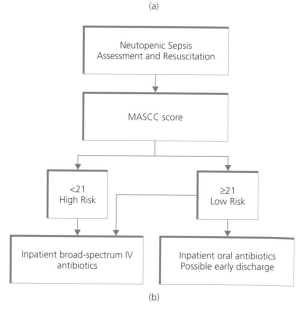

(b)

Figure 12.1 Management of low-risk neutropenic sepsis patients. (a) MASCC score. (b) Flow diagram. IV, intravenous; BP, blood pressure; COPD, chronic obstructive pulmonary disease; MASCC, Multinational Association for Supportive Care in Cancer.

prophylactically in chemotherapy regimens known to have high rates of myelosupression.

Metastatic spinal cord compression

Metastatic spinal cord compression (MSCC) is defined by the National Institute for Health and Clinical Excellence (National Institute for Health and Clinical Excellence 2008) as 'spinal cord or cauda equina compression by direct pressure and/or induction of vertebral collapse or instability by metastatic spread or direct extension of malignancy that threatens or causes neurological disability'.

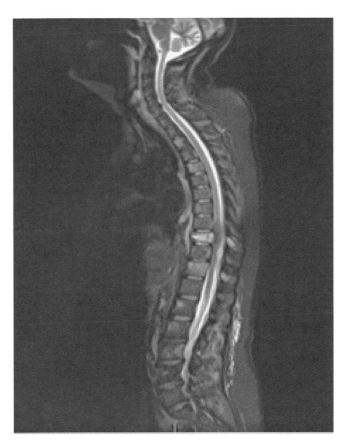

Figure 12.2 T2-weighted sagittal MRI scan demonstrating MSCC at the T9 level.

Secondary tumour deposits in the bones of the vertebrae may expand the bone or cause collapse such that there is pressure and compression of the spinal cord within the bony canal at the posterior aspect of the bone. Soft-tissue disease adjacent to the bone may have the same effect. Metastatic spinal cord compression occurs in 5–10% of cancer patients and is most commonly seen in lung, prostate and breast cancer (Figure 12.2). It is a major cause of morbidity due to pain and loss of function.

Most patients present with back pain, which as a common benign symptom makes the diagnosis challenging. Recent-onset back pain in oncology patients (especially if in the thoracic region) with a radicular (band-like) distribution or associated with neurological signs should be immediately referred for investigation. Unfortunately, the median duration from onset of pain to medical intervention is still as long as 2 months. Sensory disturbance, weakness and autonomic dysfunction are late signs and their absence should not delay investigations.

If the patient is ambulant at diagnosis, 70% will maintain this function after treatment; conversely, less than 10% of those paraplegic at diagnosis will improve. Consequently, early recognition of symptoms, diagnosis and treatment is crucial for better outcome (see Box 12.1). It is advisable that patients are managed in specialist centres where out-of-hours magnetic resonance imaging (MRI), neurosurgical and radiotherapy services are available. Patients may be treated with either surgery (see Chapter 4) or radiotherapy (see Chapter 7), or both.

Box 12.1 Management of MSCC

- **Dexamethasone::** 16 mg per day.
- Urgent whole-spine MRI (out-of-hours MRI service often required).
- **Urgent palliative radiotherapy::** five daily fractions or single fraction, depending on prognosis.
- **Neurosurgery::** indicated for spinal instability, those without a histological diagnosis or if life expectancy is more than 6 months in ambulant fit patients, especially if there is only one level of compression.
- **Chemotherapy::** started urgently for a chemosensitive tumour (e.g. germ cell tumour, lymphoma).
- Multidisciplinary rehabilitation (physiotherapy and occupational therapy).

Superior vena cava obstruction

Superior vena cava obstruction (SVCO) is caused by malignancy in 90% of cases and is typically seen in lung cancer and lymphoma. It causes dyspnoea, swelling of the face, neck and upper limbs, cough and headache. It is not an emergency condition unless associated with stridor. The diagnosis is confirmed by contrast computed tomography (CT) scan (Figure 12.3) and, in the case of a new presentation of cancer, biopsy.

Patients are usually started on dexamethasone (16 mg per day) and then considered for superior vena cava stent insertion prior to definitive treatment with radiotherapy or chemotherapy. Superior vena cava stents (Figure 12.4) relieve symptom in up to 95% of patients, compared to 77% for other modalities of treatment, and can provide immediate relief (symptoms can take up to 2 weeks to respond to radiotherapy). Chemotherapy is usually restricted to highly chemosensitive tumours such as small-cell lung cancer (SCLC), lymphoma or germ cell tumours.

Hypercalcaemia of malignancy

Malignant hypercalcaemia is a frequent complication of metastatic bone disease; however, as a paraneoplastic process it may occur

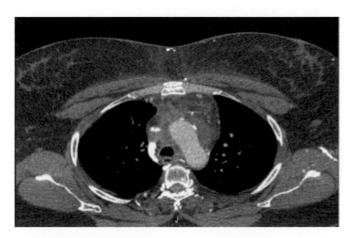

Figure 12.3 Contrast-enhanced CT thorax revealing SVCO due to mediastinal lymphadenopathy.

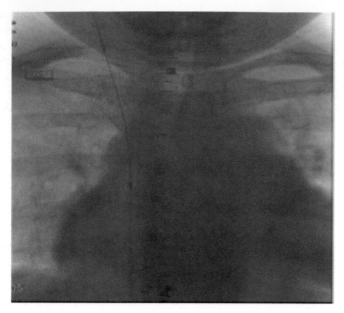

Figure 12.4 SVCO managed with stent placement to relieve obstruction. Image shows mediastinum widened by tumour and radiological guide wire for stent insertion.

in the absence of bone metastasis. It is the commonest metabolic complication of cancer, occurring in 10% of patients. It is an indicator of poor prognosis (median survival is 3–4 months and 80% die within 1 year). Although possible in any malignancy, it is most frequently associated with multiple myeloma (50% of cases), breast cancer (20%) and lung cancer (20%).

Pathophysiology of hypercalcaemia

Serum calcium levels are controlled by the parathyroid hormone (PTH) axis (Figure 12.5). Hypercalcaemia of malignancy is caused by tumour production of PTH-related peptide (PTRrP) in 80%

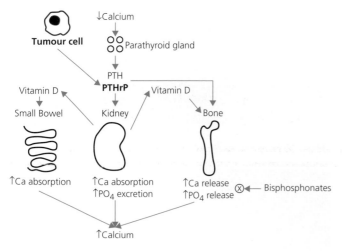

Figure 12.5 Endocrine regulation of calcium.

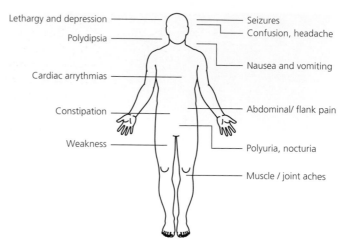

Figure 12.6 Signs and symptoms of hypercalcaemia.

of cases, while lytic bone metastases make up the majority of the remainder.

Management

Hypercalcaemia can cause multiple symptoms (Figure 12.6). Investigations should include corrected calcium, full blood count (FBC), renal and hepatic function, serum magnesium (as low magnesium is a common concurrent finding) and an electrocardiogram (ECG). Serum PTH may be helpful in patients without a known cancer diagnosis as it will be normal or low in hypercalcaemia of malignancy. Measurement of PTHrP is not routinely indicated and is not available outside specialist laboratories.

Treatment

The average patient with malignant hypercalcaemia is 4 litres in negative balance, so rehydration with 0.9% saline is central to treatment. For mild cases ($Ca^{++} < 3.0$ mmol/l), this may be all that is needed. Rehydration may provoke hypomagnesaemia and hypocalcaemia, which should be corrected as needed.

Higher calcium levels (>3.0 mmol/l) usually require bisphosphonates. Serum calcium usually begins to fall within 48 hours and normalises within 5 days. Duration of action is 3–4 weeks, so repeated treatments are normal. Refractory cases may respond to corticosteroids, calcitonin, gallium or RANK (receptor activator of nuclear factor-kB) ligand inhibitors (e.g. Denosumab), but success is variable and prognosis is frequently poor.

Lymphangitis carcinomatosis

Lymphangitis carcinomatosis refers to infiltration of the pulmonary lymphatic vasculature by tumour cells, leading to obstruction and congestion. It is associated with adenocarcinomas in 80% of cases, and is most commonly seen in breast, gastric, lung and colon cancer. Symptoms include breathlessness, dry cough and

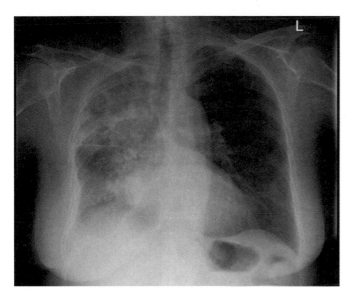

Figure 12.7 Lymphangitis carcinomatosis affecting the right lung in a patient with adenocarcinoma of the lung.

occasionally haemoptysis. Chest x-ray (CXR) findings (Figure 12.7) are absent in up to 30% of patients, in which case CT chest is diagnostic.

Anticancer therapies

The development of lymphangitis is associated with a poor prognosis. The only effective treatment is of the underlying cancer, so is restricted to chemotherapy and hormone-sensitive tumours such as SCLC and breast cancer. Radiotherapy to hilar and mediastinal lymphadenopathy may be of some benefit.

Symptom control

In many cases, lymphangitis carcinomatosis is resistant to treatment and progressively worsens, so symptom control and early palliative care involvement is vital. Opioids (e.g. oral morphine 2.5 mg 4 hourly) and/or benzodiazepines (e.g. lorazepam 0.5–1.0 mg sublingually) can provide relief from breathlessness. Although they should be used with care as they are respiratory depressants, their role is important, especially in the terminal phase of illness. Corticosteroids (e.g. dexamethasone 4 mg b.d.) are often used to reduce pulmonary congestion, although there is no evidence to support their use.

Hypomagnasaemia

Hypomagnasaemia is commonly associated with chemotherapeutic agents (e.g. cisplatin, carboplatin, cetuximab) and is exacerbated by vomiting and diarrhoea. It has potentially fatal multisystem effects (Table 12.3) and yet is still underdiagnosed.

Table 12.3 Manifestations of hypomagnesaemia.

Neuromuscular	Weakness
	Tremors
	Seizures
	Paraesthesia
	Tetany
	Chvostek sign
	Trousseau sign
	Nystagmus (horizontal and vertical)
Cardiac	Prolonged QT interval
	Ventricular tachycardia
	Ventricular fibrillation
	Enhanced digitalis toxicity
	Nonspecific T-wave changes
	Torsade de pointes
Metabolic	Hypokalaemia
	Hypocalcaemia

Table 12.4 Treatment of hypomagnaseaemia.

Severity of hypomagnasaemia	Treatment
Mild (>0.4 mmol/l) and asymptomatic	Magnesium glycerophosphate (tablet or liquid) Slow release: magnesium oxide, magnesium chloride Total: 24 mmol in 24 hours, divided doses
Moderate or severe (<0.4 mmol/l) and/ or symptomatic	5 g (20 mmol) MgSO$_4$ in 1 l normal saline over minimum 3 hours (longer infusions (8–10 hours) improve absorption) Repeat for the next 3–5 days until serum magnesium is normal If renal impairment occurs: 2.5 g (10 mmol) MgSO$_4$ over 24 hours
Emergency	In HDU/ITU setting only: 2 g MgSO$_4$ IV over 5–7 minutes* Then treat with further IV MgSO$_4$ as above

*Rapid magnesium infusions can cause cardiac arrhythmias.
HDU, high-dependency unit; ITU, intensive therapy unit; IV, intravenous.

Treatment of hypomagnasaemia

Asymptomatic patients with mild to moderate hypomagnesaemia are suitable for oral magnesium therapy (Table 12.4). This is poorly tolerated as it causes diarrhoea, so slow-release formulations are preferred if available.

Patients with moderate/severe symptomatic hypomagnesaemia require cardiac monitoring and intravenous magnesium replacement (Table 12.4). Repeated daily treatments are required as up to 50% of infused magnesium is excreted in the urine. Magnesium takes time to equilibrate in the body, so serum levels should not be checked for 48 hours after parenteral magnesium administration.

Further reading

Levack, P., Graham, J., Collie, D., Grant, R., Kidd, J., Kunkler, I. *et al.* (2002) Don't wait for sensory level – listen to symptoms: a prospective audit of the delays in diagnosis of malignant cord compression. *Clinical Oncology*, **14(6)**, 472–480.

National Cancer Action Team (2011) *National Cancer Peer Review Programme Manual for Cancer Services: Acute Oncology – Including Metatastic Spinal Cord Compression Measures*, http://www.dh.gov.uk/en /Publicationsandstatistics/Publications/PublicationsPolicyAndGuidance /DH_125727 (last accessed 8 March 2013).

National Institute for Health and Clinical Excellence (n.d.) Guidelines on the management of neutropenic sepsis, http://guidance.nice.org.uk (last accessed 8 March 2013).

National Institute for Health and Clinical Excellence (2004) Stent placement for vena caval obstruction, http://www.nice.org.uk/nicemedia/live /11137/31238/31238.pdf (last accessed 8 March 2013).

National Institute for Health and Clinical Excellence (2008) Metastatic spinal cord compression: diagnosis and management of adults at risk of and with metastatic spinal cord compression, http://www.nice.org.uk/guidance /index.jsp?action=byID&o=11648 (last accessed 8 March 2013).

Saif, M.W. (2008) Management of hypomagnesemia in cancer patients receiving chemotherapy. *Journal of Supportive Oncology*, **6(5)**, 243–248.

CHAPTER 13

Cancer in the Elderly

Alistair Ring and Juliet E. Wright

Brighton and Sussex Medical School, Royal Sussex County Hospital, Brighton, UK

OVERVIEW

- Half of all cancer diagnoses are made in men and women aged 70 and over
- The global population is ageing and the management of cancer in older patients is likely to become an increasing challenge
- Older patients are underrepresented in clinical trials
- Older patients with cancer are a heterogeneous population from physiological, social and psychological perspectives
- Assessments of health based on a Comprehensive Geriatric Assessment (CGA) may bring more objectivity to treatment decisions

The ageing population and cancer

The global population is ageing. In the UK it is estimated that the number of people aged 60 or over will increase from 12 million (21% of the population) in 1996 to 18 million (30%) by 2066 (Figure 13.1). Life expectancies have also increased, such that a 70-year-old man in the UK today is expected to live a median of 14.4 years and a 70-year-old woman 16.6 years (Table 13.1). The incidence of most tumour types increases with age, and nearly 80% of all cancer deaths occur in people aged 70 or older. In 2008, 155 000 people aged 70 or older received a cancer diagnosis, half of all of those diagnosed with cancer that year. With the ageing of the population, both the proportion of cancers diagnosed in older patients and the absolute number of cancer diagnoses in this patient group are likely to rise.

Challenges in management of older patients with cancer

Clinical trial data

Management decisions should be based on evidence from clinical trials in representative populations. However, historically older patients have been underrepresented in clinical trials. This has occurred due to upper age limits for trial entry and investigations centring around interventions that are likely to be poorly tolerated

ABC of Cancer Care, First Edition.
Edited by Carlo Palmieri, Esther Bird and Richard Simcock.
© 2013 John Wiley & Sons, Ltd. Published 2013 by John Wiley & Sons, Ltd.

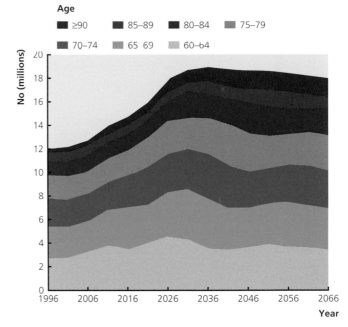

Figure 13.1 Projected numbers of people aged 60 years and over in the UK, 1996–2066. Reproduced from: Khaw K-T. How many, how old, how soon? BMJ; Nov 20: 1999:319:1350–1352. Copyright © 1999, with permission from BMJ Publishing Group Ltd.

Table 13.1 Life expectancy of men and women in the UK in 2010.

	70-year-old median survival (years)	80-year-old median survival (years)
Men	14.4	8.3
Women	16.6	9.6

or which are contraindicated in older patients due to coexistent health problems. In addition, there is often reluctance on behalf of clinicians to offer trials to older patients, and in some cases reluctance on behalf of older patients to enter clinical trials. As a result, there is a lack of data to guide many of the key treatment management decisions in this patient population.

Physiological changes in older patients

The ageing process is associated with changes in physiological reserve which may have implications for the tolerance of anticancer therapies and may mean that treatments that are routinely considered in younger patients are not appropriate or advisable in some older patients.

Cardiac function becomes less efficient with increased fibrous tissue in the muscular wall of the heart. Degenerative changes at the sinoatrial (SA) node impair the chronotropic response to stress. An increased prevalence of atherosclerosis, hypertensive changes and impaired autonomic response challenges the cardiovascular reserve of patients. Both traditional cytotoxics (such as anthracyclines) and modern targeted anticancer therapies (such as trastuzumab and bevacizumab) have potentially toxic effects on the cardiovascular system, such that their use needs to be closely monitored in older patients. Age-related changes occur in ventilation and perfusion parameters affecting respiratory function, which have implications for the management of pulmonary malignancies, particularly when radical therapies such as surgery or radical radiotherapy are being considered. Decreased bone marrow reserve is also well recognised to be associated with ageing and may result in increased toxicity with myelosuppressive therapies, such that dose modifications and the use of growth factor support may be needed.

Effects of ageing on pharmacokinetics

The complex physiological changes that occur with age are also associated with significant changes in pharmacokinetics, such that special care and consideration are required when prescribing. Muscle mass falls by 1.0–1.5% per year from the age of 40 onwards. By the age of 80, elderly individuals have lost 50% of the lean tissue they had as young adults. This change in lean mass is accompanied by a reduction in strength in healthy men and women of 1–2% per year. The reduction in lean body mass results in an increased plasma concentration and risk of toxicity for drugs distributed in muscle. With an increase in fat mass, the volume of distribution of fat-soluble drugs such as opiates increases, with significant risks of toxicity with cumulative doses. There is a decreased volume of distribution for water-soluble drugs, with subsequent increased plasma concentrations and requirement for the adjustment of loading doses of such medications. Total albumin decreases by 12–25% with age and is further depressed by heart failure, renal disease, rheumatoid arthritis, hepatic cirrhosis and malignancies, such that drug binding capacity is reduced by 12–25%, with increased free drug and further toxicity risk.

Ageing effects are also seen in drug absorption, distribution, metabolism and clearance. Reduction in the secretion of saliva and gastric acid, with decreased gastrointestinal (GI) motility and reduced splanchnic blood flow, reduces the rate of drug absorption, with an increased time taken to reach steady state. Glomerular filtration rate declines by 1% per year over the age of 40 years, with a 50% reduction in the number of functioning nephrons in a 90-year-old compared to a 40-year-old. Careful consideration of the appropriate dosing of drugs that are principally cleared by the kidney is essential. Liver volume decreases with age, with reduction in liver blood flow, such that first pass-metabolism is reduced. With a reduction in CP450 activity in the frail elderly, hepatic clearance of drugs is also reduced. The variation in individuals is significant and regimes to monitor toxicity and response must be adapted to account for this.

Nutritional status

Patient in their 80s are reported to have five times the risk of malnutrition compared to patients in their 50s. The aetiology may simply reflect the underlying malignancy, but will be further exacerbated by poor dentition, reduced appetite and nausea secondary to medications, functional and mechanical dysphagia, dyspepsia, constipation, reduced dexterity and global causes such as depression and reduced cognition. The consequences are equally diverse, including increased risk of sepsis, delayed wound healing, muscle wasting and poor mobility. An assessment of a patient's nutritional status is a vital component of the initial workup, such that management can be targeted and monitored alongside other treatment goals.

Social and neuropsychological changes

While the variation in physiological parameters makes the assessment of function challenging in elderly people, social and psychological assessment is also different in this group. With an increasing incidence of cognitive impairment and cerebrovascular disease and increased risks of delirium and depression, complications of active interventions can raise new and significant declines in function. Patient expectations are often lower, with the expectation that old age is associated with morbidity.

The multiple factors that need to be considered when managing older patients with cancer are summarised in Figure 13.2.

Variability in ageing

The multiple factors which may accompany the ageing process and thereby complicate treatment are by no means inevitable. Age itself tells us much about populations but less about individuals, and the interindividual variation in function seen in different age groups increases as patients get older. There is much literature on the use of objective measures for assessing 'true' age, with emphasis on physiological function above chronological age. Increasingly, this literature, typically the domain of elderly medicine, is being applied to the care of older patients with cancer.

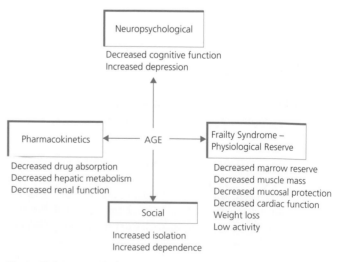

Figure 13.2 Factors which need to be taken into account when managing older patients with cancer.

Table 13.2 Components of a Comprehensive Geriatric Assessment.

Domain	Example assessment tool	Description
Comorbidity	Charlson Index	Weighted comorbidity index, score depending on presence or absence of defined comorbidities (score: 0–37)
Function	Activities of Daily Living (ADL)	Assessment of independence in six activities (score: 0–6)
	Instrumental Activities of Daily Living (IADL)	Assessment of independence in eight activities (score: 0–8)
Nutrition	Mini Nutritional Assessment (MNA)	Questionnaire and anthropometric measures; patients defined as: normal, at risk of malnutrition or malnourished (score: 0–30)
Cognition	Mini Mental State Examination (MMSE)	Questionnaire (score: 0–30)
Psychological	Geriatric Depression Score (GDS-15)	15-item questionnaire (score: 0–4 normal, 5–9 mild depression, 10–15 more severe depression)
Physical	Falls in last 6 months	
	Timed Up and Go (TUG)	Time to walk 3 m and return from sitting in a chair (score: time to complete)
Polypharmacy	Number of medications	Beer's criteria to assess appropriateness of medications
Social situation	Medical Outcomes Study (MOS) Social Support Survey	18 questions in four domains, plus one additional question

Objective assessments: Comprehensive Geriatric Assessment

A Comprehensive Geriatric Assessment (CGA) is a process that formally examines a number of domains: comorbidity, function, nutrition, cognition, psychological, physical, polypharmacy and social status (Table 13.2). Achieving a truly comprehensive assessment requires an integrated intervention from a multidisciplinary core 'firm', consisting of a specialist physiotherapist, occupational therapist, dietitian, specialist nurse, social worker and geriatrician.

The objective measures included in a CGA may prove to be valuable tools in overcoming the challenges of managing the heterogeneous population of older patients by helping to answer some key questions:

1 Is the newly diagnosed cancer likely to limit life expectancy, or do competing causes of mortality as a result of comorbidities/other health problems dominate outlook?
2 Is the patient likely to tolerate the proposed intervention: surgery, radiotherapy or chemotherapy?
3 Are there identifiable ways of improving function or fitness in order to improve treatment tolerance or quality of life?

Optimising care

The combined assessments of the multidisciplinary team (MDT) will enable an accurate assessment of the current functional and nutritional status of the patient. Treatment options can be considered from a holistic view with respect to outcomes. Appropriate interventions for functional, nutritional and psychological support can be planned for in advance and patients' expectations appropriately set, with quality of life being a key determinant in the management plan.

Such an integrated approach should ensure that the right patients get the right treatment, irrespective of age. The MDT will require time and training to ensure that patients are fully informed to choose and to consent to the treatment options available to them. The infrastructure to support this integrated care needs to be fully evidence-based, with the hospital acting as the hub for community services vital to the support of patients involved in these complex treatment regimes.

Further reading

Caillet, P., Canoui-Poitrine, F., Vouriot, J., Berle, M., Reinald, N., Krypciak, S. et al. (2011) Comprehensive geriatric assessment in the decision-making process in elderly patients with cancer: ELCAPA study. *Journal of Clinical Oncology*, **29**, 3636–3642.

Cancer Research UK (2011) Cancer incidence by age, http://info.cancer researchuk.org/cancerstats/incidence/age (last accessed 8 March 2013).

Cancer Research UK (2011) Cancer mortality by age, http://info.cancer researchuk.org/cancerstats/mortality/age (last accessed 8 March 2013).

Ellis, G., Whitehead, M.A., Robinson, D., O'Neill, D. & Langhorne, P. (2011) Comprehensive geriatric assessment for older adults admitted to hospital: meta-analysis of randomised controlled trials. *British Medical Journal*, **343**, d6553.

Lichtman, S.M., Wildiers, H., Chatelut, E., Steer, C., Budman, D., Morrison, V.A. et al. (2007) International Society of Geriatric Oncology Chemotherapy Taskforce: evaluation of chemotherapy in older patients – an analysis of the medical literature. *Journal of Clinical Oncology*, **25**, 1832–1843.

CHAPTER 14

Nutrition

Mhairi Donald

Sussex Cancer Centre, Royal Sussex County Hospital, Brighton, UK

OVERVIEW

- Many physical and psychological aspects of cancer can adversely affect nutritional status, which in turn can affect responses to treatment and quality of life
- Dietary adaptations should be implemented to help minimise specific nutritional symptoms and improve quality of life
- Patients may benefit from an individual consultation with a registered dietitian

Introduction

A healthy, balanced diet is important for everyone. However, the development of cancer and implementation of anticancer treatments can have a detrimental effect on maintaining an adequate nutritional intake and good nutritional status.

Nutritional depletion and malnutrition in the cancer patient are multifactorial:

- Metabolic changes caused by the growth of the tumour can alter the utilisation of energy.
- Physical effects of cancer, such as dysphagia in oesophageal cancer, can cause reduced nutrient intake. Patients with colorectal cancer may experience increased nutrient losses or impaired absorption.
- Side effects of anticancer treatment and anatomical effects of surgery may be pronounced and prolonged, including gastrointestinal (GI) effects, anorexia, nausea, vomiting and taste changes.
- Psychological effects of a cancer diagnosis can include sadness, anxiety and depression, which can adversely affect appetite and oral intake.

Nutritional status may change prior to a cancer diagnosis, manifesting as unintentional weight loss and malnutrition. The severity of this can be site- and stage-dependent; there are higher incidences associated with advanced disease and with sites such as the head and neck and pancreas. By the time they are diagnosed, 60% of patients with lung cancer and up to 80% of patients with stomach or oesophageal cancers will have lost weight. By contrast, cancer of the breast and prostate – particularly in the early stages of disease – are less likely to be predisposed to undernutrition.

Significant weight loss can influence performance status and suitability for cancer treatment, so early nutritional screening and management of nutritional problems is crucial. All inpatients should be screened on admission and all outpatients screened on their first appointment or if there is clinical concern (National Institute for Health and Clinical Excellence 2006). Tools such as the Malnutrition Universal Screening Tool (MUST) can be used. Alternatively, if a patient displays any of the following they will be regarded as malnourished:

- body mass index (BMI) less than 18.5 kg/m^2;
- unintentional weight loss greater than 10% within the last 3–6 months;
- BMI less than 20 kg/m^2 and unintentional weight loss greater than 5% within the last 3–6 months.

Nutritional intervention should be initiated as soon as any issues are detected. Optimising nutritional status is an important goal for any anticancer treatment. Adequate nutrition can improve tolerance and response to treatment, immune function and wound healing, reduce toxicities and complications and improve quality of life.

Surgery

Surgery has nutritional implications: there may be changes in metabolic responses triggered by a surgical trauma, as well as periods of fasting pre- and postsurgery, and delays in the return to normal food intake. Surgery itself may cause permanent anatomical changes which have an effect on nutrition (see Table 14.1). Enhanced recovery programmes in cancer surgery help support nutritional status by avoiding preoperative fasting, using preoperative carbohydrate loading and initiating early postoperative oral nutrition.

Chemotherapy and biological agents

The cytotoxic effect of chemotherapy on normal, rapidly dividing cells, particularly those in oral and intestinal mucosal, can lead to common side effects impacting on nutritional intake (e.g. sore

ABC of Cancer Care, First Edition.
Edited by Carlo Palmieri, Esther Bird and Richard Simcock.
© 2013 John Wiley & Sons, Ltd. Published 2013 by John Wiley & Sons, Ltd.

Table 14.1 Surgical procedures and subsequent nutritional issues.

Site	Surgical procedure	Nutritional issues	Nutritional management
Brain	Tumour removal or debulking	High levels of steroid may cause excessive weight gain	Healthy eating Use of healthy snacks
Head and neck	Partial or total glossectomy Pharyngolaryngectomy Mandibulectomy Transoral laser surgery	Surgical resection may restrict or completely prevent the patient's ability to consume food orally Denture may no longer be suitable, requiring refitting	Food texture change Food fortification Supplementation of intake with oral nutritional supplements Gastrostomy tube feeding
Oesophageal	Oesophageal resection Partial or total oesophagectomy or oesophagogastrectomy	Early satiety Nausea Reflux Stricture of anastomosis may cause dysphagia Dumping syndrome	Postoperative jejunostomy tube feeding Food texture change Supplementation of intake with oral nutritional supplements Small, frequent meals and snacks Avoidance of drinks with meals
Stomach	Subtotal or total gastrectomy	Small-stomach syndrome Dumping syndrome Malabsorption Anaemia	Postoperative jejunostomy tube feeding Food texture change Supplementation of intake with oral nutritional supplements Small, frequent meals and snacks Avoidance of drinks with meals Vitamin B12 injections
Pancreas	Pancreaticoduodenectomy	Fat malabsorption May develop diabetes mellitus	Commencement of enzyme supplements Expert advice on fat and simple carbohydrate intake
Lung	Lobectomy	Fatigue Early satiety	Small, frequent meals and snacks Food fortification
Breast	Local excision or mastectomy	Postsurgery, may be at risk of lymphodema	Healthy eating Use of healthy snacks Avoidance of weight gain during the first year post diagnosis
Gynaecological cancers	May require resection or diversion of nongynaecological organs Peritoneal debulking	Formation of ileostomy, colostomy and/or urostomy	Adequate fluids Small, frequent meals and snacks Mixed, healthy diet
Colorectal	Bowel resection	Formation of ileostomy or colostomy	Adequate fluids Mixed, healthy diet

mouth) (see Chapter 6). These are sometimes referred to as 'nutrition impact symptoms'. Patients will often experience clusters of nutrition impact symptoms. A number of symptoms are associated with increased levels of malnutrition, including nausea, reduced appetite, taste changes, mucositis, oesophagitis and alteration in bowel habits.

Radiotherapy

Despite improvements in targeting radiation, patients still experience site-specific side effects as a result of damage to associated healthy tissue. The addition of concurrent chemotherapy is likely to increase early toxicity and affect nutritional status (see Table 14.2). Radiotherapy is delivered daily, over periods ranging from one session to up to 5 days a week for 7 weeks, and may require considerable journey time to radiotherapy facilities. This impacts on activities of daily living, including shopping, food preparation/cooking and timing of meals – all of which are barriers to patients achieving sufficient oral intake.

Nutritional goals

The goals of nutrition intervention will be tailored to the diagnosis and prognosis of the patient and their management plan, and may change over time. Improving nutritional status during treatment may be difficult, so the goal of treatment might be to simply maintain weight and nutritional status. Identifying and actively managing the nutrition impact symptoms through the cancer journey is vital.

General energy requirements are:

- 30–35 kcal (kg body weight (BW)/day) for ambulant patients;
- 20–25 kcals (kg BW/day) for bed-bound patients (Arends et al. 2006).

Poor appetite

Poor appetite is the most commonly reported problem in cancer patients, followed by early satiety (feeling full quickly). Poor appetite arises as a result of the biological effects of cancer and treatment side effects. Patients often report consuming smaller portions.

Table 14.2 Radiotherapy side effects and their management.

Targeted tumour	Organs/cells damaged	Associated nutrition impact symptoms	Medical management	Dietary management
Mouth, throat, head and neck	Mucosal epithelium Taste buds Salivary glands	Pain, mucositis, loss of taste, change in taste, xerostomia (dry mouth), dysphagia, trismus, dehydration	Gelclair MuGard™ Benzdyamine spray or rinse Pain control	Change in texture to soft, moist, semisolid or liquid Use of oral nutritional supplements Enteral tube/gastrostomy feeding
Upper GI tract—oesophagus	Oesophagus Stomach	Oesophagitis, epigastric pain, dysphagia, indigestion, early satiety	Pain control Sucralfate Antacids	Change in texture to soft, moist, semisolid or liquid Use of oral nutritional supplements Enteral tube feeding
Lung	Oesophagus Stomach	Oesophagitis, epigastric pain, dysphagia, indigestion, dyspnoea, early satiety	Pain control Sucralfate Antacids	Small, frequent, nutrient-dense meals Change in texture to soft, moist, semisolid or liquid Use of oral nutritional supplements
Cervix, endometrial, prostate, bladder, colorectal, anus	Small intestine Large intestine Bladder	Diarrhoea, abdominal cramps, cystitis, dehydration	Antidiarrhoeal Antispasmodic Pain control	Adequate fluid intake, mixed balanced diet Elemental diets, low-fat and low-lactose diets show some benefit on treat and for late effects (only to be undertaken with dietetic supervision) No evidence for fibre restriction during treatment, which can be unnecessarily restrictive Late effects may also benefit from a restriction of oligo-, di-, mono saccharides and polyols under dietetic supervision

Evidence suggests that patients who eat more frequently have a higher intake, so they should be actively encouraged to eat small, frequent meals and between-meal snacks. They should also be encouraged to use or add foods that are more nutrient dense weight for weight, to maximise the amount of nutrients in a small volume (e.g. full cream milk, cheese and yoghurt). See Box 14.1 for a sample menu.

Other anticipated symptoms will benefit from individualised medical management, but may also benefit from specific dietary support (see Table 14.3). Intensive nutritional counselling delivered by dietitians has been shown to minimise weight loss and deterioration in nutritional status, physical functioning and quality of life.

Oral nutritional supplements

Oral nutritional supplements (ONS) may help increase the nutrient intake of patients. There are a range of ONS available, produced by a variety of companies. They can be prescribed in accordance with the Advisory Committee on Borderline Substances (ACBS). Generally, these supplements are used in addition to normal foods when a patient is not fully meeting their requirements. They include a variety of styles and flavours (see Figure 14.1):

- milkshake-style drinks;
- fruit juice-style drinks;
- yoghurt-style drinks;
- soups;
- desserts;
- fresh milk mixes.

Table 14.3 Symptoms impacting on nutritional intake and first-line management.

Taste changes

Taste changes are positively correlated with a decrease in dietary intake. There are five basic tastes: sweet, bitter, sour, salt and umami (the savouriness of protein-rich foods). Changes in the threshold of these basic tastes can result in:

- a reduction in taste sensitivity (hypogeusia)
- an absence of taste sensation, where food is tasteless (ageusia)
- a distortion of normal taste, where food tastes bitter or metallic (dysgeusia)

Taste changes may result from:

- the cancer itself (particularly common in advanced cancer)
- radiotherapy, particularly to the head and neck (causes a destructive effect on the sensory organs, oral cavity, salivary glands, tongue and the nerves associated with taste perception)
- chemotherapy (altered taste and smell reported in up to 75% of those receiving chemotherapy)
- malnutrition
- ageing
- poor oral hygiene, infection or dry mouth

Red meat is often associated with a metallic/bitter taste (possibly due to high iron content). Use alternative sources of protein, fish, poultry, eggs, cheese, soya and dairy produce. Marinating meat with fruit juice, wine, cider or beer may help

Add soups, sauces and plenty of seasonings, especially herbs and spices, to savoury dishes

Ensure good oral hygiene

Encourage serving of foods at room temperature or chilled

Dry mouth (Xerostomia)

Dry mouth is a commonly reported nutrition impact symptom. Lack of or reduction in saliva can make chewing and swallowing difficult and effortful. This may occur as a result of:

- the cancer itself
- damage to the salivary glands as a result of surgery or radiotherapy
- chemotherapy and other medications

Ensure meals are moist through the use of extra gravy, sauces, cream, and butter

Avoid very dry foods such as biscuits, crackers and bread

Sip on liquids throughout the day

Rinse the mouth frequently with bicarbonate of soda solution (1 tsp. of soda in half a litre of water)

Offer dry mouth products and/or artificial saliva

Nausea and vomiting

Nausea and vomiting occur in up to 44% of patients

They commonly occur as a result of chemotherapy or pain-relieving drugs

They can result from diseases in the abdomen or GI tract

Patients should have individual drug-management plans that are regularly reviewed

Encourage small, frequent meals, with between-meal snacks

Cold or room-temperature foods may be easier to tolerate

Dry biscuits, particularly first thing in the morning, may help

Avoid fried, greasy and spicy foods, which may upset the stomach

Ginger-containing products can be helpful (e.g. ginger ale/beer, ginger biscuits)

Foods such as ice lollies, sorbets and ice cubes in a fizzy drink can be easier to take and are refreshing

Dysphagia

Difficulty in swallowing may occur as result of:

- cancer causing physical obstructions, e.g. with an oesophageal cancer (the insertion of an oesophageal stent can palliate this)
- Surgical removal of the cancer where it affects the anatomic ability to eat (e.g. removal of part of the tongue or palate)
- Radiation- or chemotherapy-induced mucositis
- Oesophagitis caused by radiotherapy, particularly to the oesophagus and lung

A formal swallow assessment by a speech and language therapist may suggest a change in diet consistency and swallowing techniques

Change food texture to soft, moist, mashable or pureed foods. It is vital that the change in texture does not compromise the nutritional value

Avoid breads, cakes, biscuits and pastries, if possible. Before eating them, soak in milk, juice, gravy or sauce

A commercially prepared oral nutritional supplement (ONS) may be required to ensure nutritional adequacy

Ensure adequate pain control and good oral care

Constipation

Some drugs (particularly pain-control drugs) can cause constipation; this may be aggravated by a reduction or change in normal oral intake. Normally, an increase in fibre-containing foods would be recommended; however, where patients are already struggling to maintain an oral intake, this may not be possible. Encouraging consumption of fibres that are easier to manage may be a better compromise

A suitable laxative should be prescribed to resolve and manage the problem

Encourage intake of 8–10 cups of fluid per day. Include water, fruit juices (including prune juice), lemon squash, fizzy drinks and soup

Eat small, frequent meals and snacks

Gentle exercise every day helps keep the bowels working

Encourage manageable sources of fibre:

- Porridge, Weetabix
- Peas, beans, lentils in a soup or stew
- Stewed, tinned fruit or mashed banana
- Vegetables added to stews, soups and casseroles

Diarrhoea

Diarrhoea can be caused by chemotherapy, pelvic radiotherapy, infection or medication, or may occur as a result of disease in the abdomen or GI tract. It can lead to dehydration and weakness

Encourage a good fluid intake of 8–10 cups of fluid per day. Include water, lemon squash, fizzy or still drinks, fruit juice, clear soups and/or Oxo or Bovril

Avoid foods and drinks that might irritate the bowel (e.g. fatty, fried or spicy foods, alcohol)

Eat little and often, with between-meal snacks

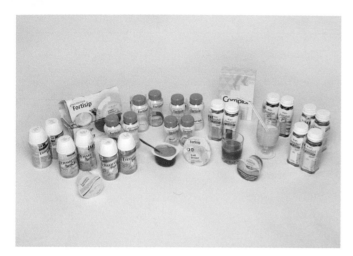

Figure 14.1 ONS from various manufacturers in a variety of preparations and formulations.

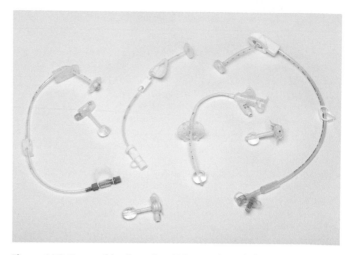

Figure 14.2 Range of feeding tubes. Tubes can be radiologically or endoscopically placed and are available in a range of lengths.

Nutritionally complete supplements, providing adequate protein, energy, vitamins and minerals, can be used as a sole source of nutrition. A dietetic referral will help to assess the appropriateness of initiating ONS and help with implementation strategies and monitoring.

Vitamin and minerals

There is a lack of evidence concerning cancer patients' requirements for micronutrients. In the case of reduced food intake and/or limited food choices, the use of a multivitamin mineral supplement administered in doses based on recommended daily amounts can be considered.

Enteral tube feeding

Tube feeding may be considered where a patient is unable to meet their nutritional intake orally as a result of surgery, or where the effects of treatments have temporarily affected the patient's ability to maintain an oral intake (e.g. chemoradiotherapy to the head and neck or upper oesophagus). Enteral feeding tubes are predominantly placed into the stomach or jejunum via the nasal route or radiologically or endoscopically placed directly into the stomach as gastrostomy tubes are placed. Gastrostomy tubes may be placed prophylactically when it is predicted there will be a high impact of treatment on nutritional status (see Figure 14.2).

Parenteral nutrition

The role of parenteral nutrition (PN; feeding via a central catheter) in cancer patients remains controversial and requires management by a specialist team. Its use should be restricted to those who do not have a functioning GI tract or where access can't be gained for enteral feeding. In advanced cancer PN requires careful consideration, those patients with an acceptable performance status and quality of life will gain the most benefit.

Weight gain

Some patients will unintentionally gain weight during treatment. Weight gain can be a result of excessive energy intake (sometimes associated with concomitant steroids), decreased physical activity and/or hormone treatments. Patients with hormone-dependent cancers such as breast and prostate cancer are often more predisposed to obesity and are at particularly high risk of gaining weight. This group should be encouraged to eat healthily and manage their weight. Weight control and exercise can markedly reduce the risk or recurrence (particularly in breast cancer) and help guard against other longer-term conditions such as heart disease, diabetes and osteoporosis

Further reading

Arends, J., Bodoky, G., Bozzetti, F., Fearon, K., Muscaritoli, M., Selga, G. *et al.* (2006) ESPEN guidelines on enteral nutrition: non-surgical oncology. *Clinical Nutrition,* **25**(2), 245–259.

National Institute for Health and Clinical Excellence (2006) *Nutrition Support in Adults: Oral Nutritional Support, Enteral Tube Feeding and Parenteral Nutrition.* National Collaborating Centre for Acute Care, London.

Shaw, C. (2011) *Nutrition and Cancer.* Blackwell, Oxford.

CHAPTER 15

Complementary and Alternative Medicine in Cancer Patients

Richard Simcock and Sarah Cavilla

Sussex Cancer Centre, Royal Sussex County Hospital, Brighton, UK

OVERVIEW

- Complementary and alternative medicine (CAM) consists of a wide-ranging and disparate group of therapies
- These therapies lack a strong evidence base and there is largely no mandatory regulation or training for therapists
- There is a high prevalence of CAM use by cancer patients, and therapies are often provided within the context of conventional medicine
- Accumulating a satisfactory evidence base is complicated by problems with methodology
- In addition to observed benefits, there is the potential for harm and drug interactions
- Patients may seek advice and support from their medical team in their choice and use of CAM

Box 15.1 **Definitions**

- **Complementary medicine** is used in addition to and alongside conventional cancer management. It is often used by patients to make them feel better or to improve side effects from their cancer or treatment. An example is aromatherapy.
- **Alternative medicine** refers to therapeutic systems and viewpoints about health that differ from those taught and practised by registered medical practitioners. An example is Chinese herbal medicine.
- **Integrated medicine** is a newer term reflecting the incorporation of more CAM therapies within the conventional medicine environment, such as acupuncture. It is a controversial term, often rejected by those who object to CAM's relative lack of evidence or scientific basis.

Background

Complementary and alternative medicines (CAMs) are therapeutic and diagnostic disciplines that exist largely outside the institutions where conventional health care is taught and provided. Increasingly, CAM is sought by cancer patients and provided in cancer treatment units. For this reason, many CAM practitioners prefer the term 'integrated medicine' (Box 15.1). The theories underpinning CAM may derive from historic, empiric or traditional models of health not shared in modern scientific medical teaching. CAM is used across a wide range of health states and is often advocated by its practitioners for use in maintaining health in the already healthy.

Exact data is difficult to obtain, but there are estimates of almost 6 million people in the UK using CAM, and in 2007 £191 million was spent on treatments (a 32% rise over 5 years), according to market research. Cancer can be a great financial challenge through loss of income and the costs to individuals for treatment can be high.

There is great demand for CAM use in cancer patients and capacity is provided by charitable and voluntary donations and the private sector. In some regions of the NHS, specific CAMs may be funded. Reports frequently suggest higher rates of CAM use in patients with cancer compared with other disease types. Depending on the definition used, estimates suggest that around a third of cancer patients use some form of CAM.

There are many factors that may cause patients to seek CAM (Box 15.2), but it is recognised that younger patients, females and those with higher education are more likely to use CAM than their counterparts.

Box 15.2 **Reasons why cancer patients may use CAM**

- To manage side effects of the cancer or the treatment (commonly pain, feeling sick, hot flushes, depression and fatigue).
- To improve their well being/relaxation.
- A belief in 'supporting the immune system' (in this context the immune system is variably defined).
- To do all they can to combat the disease.
- To feel more in control of their health: asserting a 'locus of control'.
- To address their personal beliefs.
- Their cultural background (e.g. in Africa 80% of primary health care is traditional medicine).
- Fatal relativism: If conventional treatment cannot help then there is 'nothing to lose'.

ABC of Cancer Care, First Edition.
Edited by Carlo Palmieri, Esther Bird and Richard Simcock.
© 2013 John Wiley & Sons, Ltd. Published 2013 by John Wiley & Sons, Ltd.

Table 15.1 Grouping of CAM therapies by the House of Lords Science and Technology Select Committee (2000).

Group 1	Therapies with professional organisations and training standards	Acupuncture, chiropractic, osteopathy, herbal medicine and homeopathy
Group 2	Harmless enough to complement conventional treatment	Aromatherapy, hypnotherapy and reflexology
Group 3	Scientifically unproven and unregulated	Ayurveda, crystal therapy, naturopathy, traditional Chinese medicine, iridology and kinesiology

Regulation

CAM is not professionally regulated in the UK in the same way as conventional medicine. A white paper on UK regulation was tabled in 2011 and the General Regulatory Council for Complementary Therapies (GRCCT) was established. Many societies of CAM practitioners encourage voluntary registration (e.g. the British Acupuncture Council) but there is no requirement to do so. The House of Lords' Committee groups CAMs according to safety and regulation (see Table 15.1).

Herbal medicines are not regulated or licensed. Nor is there a system of quality assurance. When buying substances from unlicensed sources, there is no guarantee that the substances are genuine or tested to be safe.

Evidence

Provision of CAM is controversial, mainly due to a lack of either strong evidence or a scientific basis. There are many problems in producing an evidence base (Box 15.3). This has prompted a government select committee review of the provision of homeopathy

---

Box 15.3 Problems with providing an evidence base in CAM

- Existing data include patients with multiple conditions of variable definition (not just cancer).
- Research is often based on effectiveness rather than efficacy; subjects obtain benefit, but not under tightly controlled circumstances.
- There is difficulty in establishing appropriate controls, e.g. 'sham' needles in acupuncture trials may produce an effect.
- There is a lack of research infrastructure and training amongst CAM practitioners.
- Funding is often not available to conduct rigorous testing in accordance with modern research governance.
- The underlying principles of therapy run counter to modern scientific thinking and as such therapists may resist what they consider a reductive scientific approach.
- Successful outcomes sought by therapists and patients are not easily measurable as they are often subjective ('well being', 'restoring balance', etc.).
- Techniques and traditions often resist standardisation, with therapies often 'tailored' to individuals. 'Dose' and duration vary from patient to patient.

---

within the NHS and many criticisms of the provision and teaching of CAM in universities.

Therapies

The most commonly offered CAM therapies are acupuncture, massage and manipulation techniques, chiropractic, aromatherapy, homeopathy and Chinese and herbal medicines.

Acupuncture

Acupuncture is a discipline of traditional Chinese medicine (TCM) in which fine needles are placed at specific points in the body believed to be connected by channels known as meridians, with the aim of correcting imbalances in the flow of energy-like qi (pronounced 'chee'). Each meridian is linked to an organ system. Abnormal flow of qi is thought to lead to disease states. When used as part of TCM, acupuncture is often accompanied by a diagnosis examining pulse characteristics and the appearance of the tongue (see Figure 15.1). TCM acupuncture is often co-prescribed with herbal medicines.

Western medical acupuncture is an adapted system widely used in modern medicine (particularly in pain clinics). It shares with TCM the naming system of points but has a more pragmatic approach to point selection and does not use herbs.

Auricular acupuncture (needling the ear) is more commonly used in TCM than in Western medical acupuncture teaching (see Figure 15.2).

Needles may be manipulated to increase the likelihood of a response. Manipulation can include transcutaneous electrical stimulation or burning substances on the needle (moxibustion).

Evidence

Acupuncture has a large evidence base, although it is typically mixed. The STandards for Reporting Interventions in Controlled Trials of Acupuncture (STRICTA) have been introduced to standardise methodologies and improve the quality of future research. Needling may release neurotransmitters, and the technique has a role in managing neuropathic pain. Some randomised trials have shown an improvement specifically in cancer-related pain in those patients receiving acupuncture when compared to placebo.

Several studies report that acupuncture improves hot flushes in women with breast cancer on hormonal treatment, at a level equivalent to drug treatment, but with a longer duration and less side effects. It may also reduce the dry mouth caused by radiation in head and neck cancer patients.

Studies demonstrate benefit in acute post-chemotherapy vomiting with concomitant antiemetic use.

Common uses

Stress, pain, nausea and vomiting, hot flushes, fatigue, xerostomia (dry mouth).

Cautions

Occasional bleeding and tenderness. Small risk of infection.

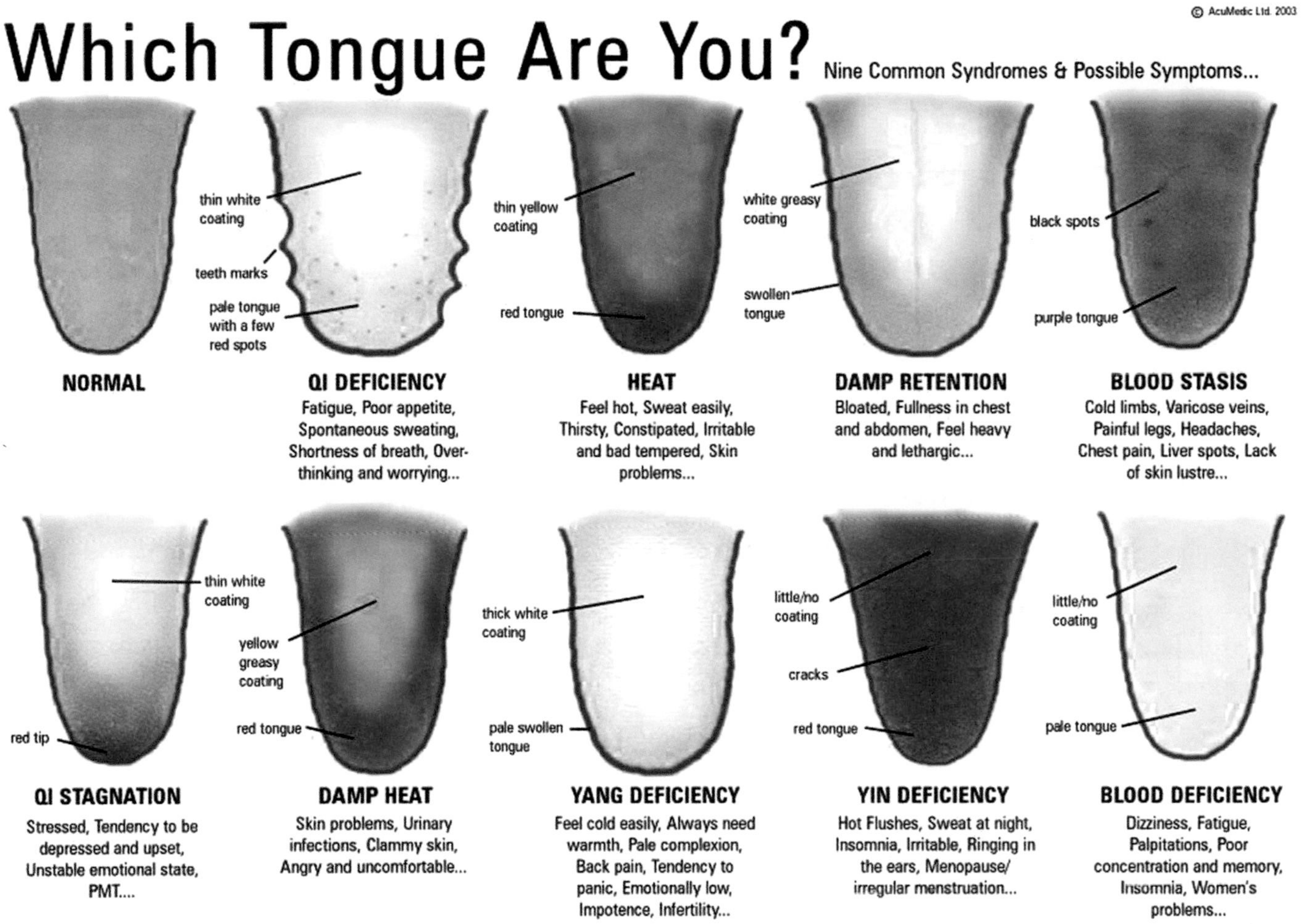

Which Tongue Are You? Nine Common Syndromes & Possible Symptoms...

© AcuMedic Ltd. 2003

NORMAL
- thin white coating
- teeth marks
- pale tongue with a few red spots

QI DEFICIENCY
Fatigue, Poor appetite, Spontaneous sweating, Shortness of breath, Over-thinking and worrying...

HEAT
- thin yellow coating
- red tongue

Feel hot, Sweat easily, Thirsty, Constipated, Irritable and bad tempered, Skin problems...

DAMP RETENTION
- white greasy coating
- swollen tongue

Bloated, Fullness in chest and abdomen, Feel heavy and lethargic...

BLOOD STASIS
- black spots
- purple tongue

Cold limbs, Varicose veins, Painful legs, Headaches, Chest pain, Liver spots, Lack of skin lustre...

QI STAGNATION
- thin white coating
- red tip

Stressed, Tendency to be depressed and upset, Unstable emotional state, PMT....

DAMP HEAT
- yellow greasy coating
- red tongue

Skin problems, Urinary infections, Clammy skin, Angry and uncomfortable...

YANG DEFICIENCY
- thick white coating
- pale swollen tongue

Feel cold easily, Always need warmth, Pale complexion, Back pain, Tendency to panic, Emotionally low, Impotence, Infertility...

YIN DEFICIENCY
- little/no coating
- cracks
- red tongue

Hot Flushes, Sweat at night, Insomnia, Irritable, Ringing in the ears, Menopause/irregular menstruation...

BLOOD DEFICIENCY
- little/no coating
- pale tongue

Dizziness, Fatigue, Palpitations, Poor concentration and memory, Insomnia, Women's problems...

Figure 15.1 Chart showing different tongue appearances used in diagnosis in TCM. Reproduced from www.acumedic.com with permission from AcuMedic Ltd.

Massage and manipulation techniques

Massage is the manipulation of skin, superficial and deep tissues. It aims to promote good health, relieve tension and encourage relaxation, and has been used for centuries worldwide. Deep-tissue massage is used in conventional cancer care in physiotherapy and as part of lymphoedema management after breast cancer axillary surgery. There are many different techniques, focusing on different anatomical locations (reflexology, hands and feet, Indian head massage), with different tools (elbows, herbal oils, stones) and numerous practices (types of manipulation: kneading, sweeping strokes, etc.). Massage can improve blood flow and lower the heart rate, promoting relaxation. Many NHS cancer departments and hospices offer massage services to patients and staff. Some massage therapists have raised concern that massage may facilitate spread of cancer, but there is no evidence that this is the case.

Evidence

Some studies show subjective benefits in anxiety, nausea, sleep and to a lesser extent pain in cancer patients. Studies have failed to confirm the specific claims of reflexology that certain 'trigger points' relate directly to distant organ systems.

Common uses

Stress, depression, anxiety, lymphoedema, psychological distress, pain, fatigue.

Cautions

Local bruising and tenderness is possible. It is recommended that direct massage of tumours be avoided. Recently irradiated skin is fragile and sensitive (see Chapter 8) and massage oils and the friction of the technique may irritate.

Chiropractic

Chiropractic is a manipulation technique that, unlike massage, is concerned with the skeleton as well as soft tissue. 'Realignment' of the skeleton is believed to enhance patient well being. There are no conclusive trials to support the use of chiropractic in cancer patients. An older meta-analysis reported benefit in lower back pain not specific to malignancy, but this has not been reproduced in more recent reviews. The techniques employed may be dangerous in patients with skeletal metastases. Chiropractic (and osteopathy), unlike all other treatments described in this chapter, is regulated by law.

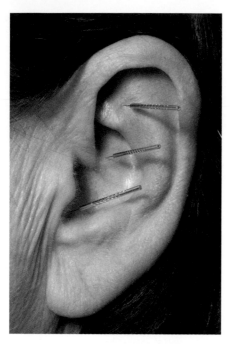

Figure 15.2 Auricular acupuncture needles, placed to improve dry mouth after radiation treatment.

Aromatherapy

Aromatherapy is the use of aromatic compounds derived from plants or from oils, which evaporate. These substances are administered by inhalation, diffusion in air or topical application, often by massage. The intent may be achieved through stimulation of the brain's olfactory (smell) and limbic system (memory and mood) and the direct effect of the plant material. Some aromatherapy products have antiseptic properties, such as tea tree and eucalyptus. Substances are selected according to the patient's mood state or desired outcome.

Evidence

There is data describing short-term benefit in anxiety and mood in cancer patients when aromatherapy is used with massage. Case studies describe an improvement in unpleasant tumour-associated smells and a role in encouraging wound healing with certain oils.

Common uses

Low mood, stress, offensive odours from tumour discharge/necrosis.

Cautions

Skin sensitivity, stinging at point of application, photo-irritation. Some substances are toxic if taken internally. The therapist should check the allergy status of the patient first.

Homeopathy

Homeopathy uses 'remedies' based on the 'law of similars': 'let like be cured by like'. Remedies are created by sequentially diluting a substance with water and agitation, termed 'potentiation', resulting in an extremely diluted mixture, which may not contain any of the original material. The NHS continues to provide homeopathy in some areas despite a government health committee concluding that it is 'medically unproven'.

Chinese and herbal medicines

Despite a long history of accumulated experience, there is no currently published robust evidence to support a clinical benefit of Chinese medicine in cancer patients, although it does have some biological rationale from laboratory-based work. There are suggestions within the data that these medicines may help toxicity secondary to cancer treatment. Limited data in colorectal cancer show that comcomitant administration of huanggi (a Chinese herb; *Astragalus propinquus*, 黄芪) with chemotherapy results in a decrease in nausea, improved leucopaenia rates and a rise in T lymphocytes.

Many of the active ingredients within herbs used in TCM can be demonstrated *in vitro* to have biological effect, usually at very high molecular dosages. The dosage and purity within individual prescriptions cannot be guaranteed without quality control or regulation.

Adverse effects reported in the use of Chinese medicine include allergy, neuropathy, liver and kidney failure.

Mistletoe

Mistletoe is a specific herbal medicine derived from the school of anthroposophy ('like will cure like'). In this instance, the parasitic nature of the mistletoe plant is thought to be similar to the relationship of tumour to host. Mistletoe is frequently used in Europe (especially Germany). Around €23 million (£16 million; USD30 million) is spent on the preparation annually. There is *in vitro* evidence suggesting that the plant may be active against cancer cells, but the 16 randomised trials published to date have been of insufficient quality to substantiate these claims. It may be administered intravenously, orally, subcutaneously or homeopathically.

Unintended effects

Herbal medicines and nutritional supplements may interact with conventional medicines: vitamins A, C and E, selenium and co-enzyme Q10 may lessen the effects of certain chemotherapies. Cranberry juice, St John's wort, *Ginkgo biloba* and co-enzyme Q10 may all interact adversely with warfarin treatment. It is important to enquire about patients' use of CAM as many surveys suggest patients will not routinely disclose their usage.

CAM used to relieve menopausal effects of breast cancer therapy may have unintended negative effects. The National Institute of Health and Clinical Excellence (NICE) recommends that women avoid soy (isoflavone), red clover, black cohosh and vitamin E, due to concern that these may stimulate oestrogen receptors within tumour cells. This risk is considered theoretical and there are no studies which confirm harm from these treatments.

Spirituality

Some therapists practise interventions and meditations aimed at bringing 'harmony' to mind and body. Some surveys of CAM include prayer within their definitions as an intervention, without scientific evidence or basis. Reiki employs a spiritual element in an adaptation of Buddhism that is less than 100 years old. Systematic reviews have found no evidence of objective benefit.

The Internet

The Internet is a massive source of information about CAM. Much online content polarises the debate around CAM with adversarial

---

Box 15.4 **Important points to consider**

- Always ask patients whether they are using any alternative or complementary medications.
- Why are they taking them? Is there a side effect that is difficult to alleviate/especially distressing?
- Is there evidence of benefit with this approach?
- What are the risks associated with this approach?
- Does the therapy have adverse effects or interact with conventional treatment?
- Is the practitioner voluntarily registered with a professional organisation?
- What experience/training does the practitioner have? Can they provide testimonial?
- Will the practitioner share details of their treatment/intervention with the medical team and vice versa?
- Will the therapy present a financial burden to the patient?
- If unsure, advise using reliable resources to research a therapy, such as hospital medicines information, pharmacists and the National Center for Complementary and Alternative Medicine (NCCAN).

---

views. Many websites are unregulated, and information may be misrepresented. Patients are advised to check more dramatic claims. It is against UK law (the 1939 Cancer Act) to advertise that a CAM can cure cancer.

Advising cancer patients

Patients should be encouraged to share their plans with their treating team and to be as fully informed as possible before starting a new therapy (as would be expected with conventional treatment). Practitioners who hold current registration with the GRCCT are seen as meeting the NHS National Cancer Action Team criteria relating to patient safety (see Box 15.4). Most hospital pharmacies provide medical information, and they can often give detailed information specific to a CAM treatment.

Further reading

Cancer Research UK (n.d.) Finding further information on complementary and alternative therapies, http://cancerhelp.cancerresearchuk.org /about-cancer/treatment/complementary-alternative/finding-further-information-on-complementary-and-alternative-therapies (last accessed 8 March 2013).

General Regulatory Council for Complementary Therapies Web site, www.grcct.org.

National Cancer Institute (n.d.) Thinking about complementary and alternative medicine: a guide for people with cancer, http://www.cancer.gov /cancertopics/cam/thinking-about-CAM (last accessed 8 March 2013).

National Center for Complementary and Alternative Medicine Web site, nccam.nih.gov.

Zollman, C., Vickers, A.J. & Richardson, J. (eds) (2008) *ABC of Complementary Medicine*, 2nd edn. Wiley-Blackwell/BMJ Books, Chichester.

CHAPTER 16

Specialist Nursing Care

Clare Sullivan, Beverley Longhurst, Amelia Cook, Elizabeth Bowman, and Jean Rodell

The Harley Street Clinic (HCA International), London, UK

OVERVIEW

- The cancer nurse's role has expanded to involve advocacy, support and information giving in addition to aspects of physical care. Such clinical nurse specialists (CNSs) in cancer are also normally a patient's nominated 'key worker'
- Patients with access to a CNS have a more favourable experiences of care
- There are nearly 3000 CNSs in the UK, with a majority specialising in breast, colorectal and urological cancers
- CNSs not only improve parts of the care pathway but also may replace traditional models of care, for example in providing follow up

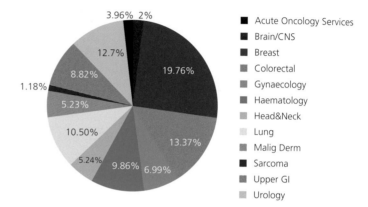

Figure 16.1 Percentage of CNS workforce by area of practice. Taken from National Cancer Action Team (2010).

Introduction

As cancer care has become more complex it has become essential to provide support and advocacy in order to enable patients and carers to more easily navigate cancer treatment and follow up. This expert support is now most often provided by nurses with specialist cancer experience, called clinical nurse specialists (CNSs; other titles include 'nurse consultant' and 'advanced nurse practitioner').

CNSs are used in 84% of trusts in England, with nearly 3000 CNSs spread across the 28 Cancer Networks. Approximately a third of these are supported by the cancer charity Macmillan. Provision varies from one whole-time-equivalent CNS for every 56 new cases of cancer to one per every 233 new cases.

A CNS will have a wide range of skills, expertise and specialist knowledge. Many CNSs have at least 10 years' experience in their field of practice (Royal College of Nurses 2005). This ensures the best possible care and support for patients and their families throughout their cancer journey. Most CNSs will specialise in a specific cancer type, which requires special education and training, and provision across different cancer types varies (see Figure 16.1). In England, the largest group of CNSs is in breast cancer (19%), followed by colorectal (14%) and urological (12%). A CNS will have a variety of roles according to specialty site, although there are core common values (see Box 16.1).

ABC of Cancer Care, First Edition.
Edited by Carlo Palmieri, Esther Bird and Richard Simcock.
© 2013 John Wiley & Sons, Ltd. Published 2013 by John Wiley & Sons, Ltd.

Box 16.1 Functions of the CNS (adapted from National Cancer Action Team 2010)

- Using knowledge of cancer and treatment to oversee and coordinate services, personalise 'the cancer pathway' for individual patients and families and meet their information needs.
- Acting as the key accessible professional for the multidisciplinary team (MDT). Proactive case management to reduce the risk to patients from disease or treatments.
- Using empathy and knowledge to assess and alleviate the psychosocial suffering of cancer, including referring to other agencies as appropriate.
- Using knowledge and insight from patients to lead service redesign in order to implement improvements and make services responsive to patient need.

In recognising the importance of patient support, the UK peer review process expects a CNS to be a core member of the multidisciplinary team (MDT) (see Chapter 1).

Emotional support

The CNS may be first introduced to the patient during the initial diagnostic pathway, when there is a suspected cancer (this is commonly the case in breast cancer). In other cancers, the CNS may first meet the patient when they are informed of their cancer diagnosis, in a consultation which will include breaking the bad news. This allows the CNS to witness the impact of and reaction to the news and then to provide support as appropriate. This support is considered so valuable that CNS presence at 'breaking bad news' is now an audited benchmark for cancer services in England.

A CNS can spend time with a patient and their family to help them begin to deal with raw and unfamiliar emotions. Emotional responses will vary, and can include shock, fear, disbelief, anger and optimism. A CNS aims to acknowledge and respect these feelings and to explore their causes. Through listening, supporting and advising, the CNS attempts to facilitate a clearer and more positive perspective for the patient.

Each patient will have individual needs, which will vary and become more obvious as the CNS–patient relationship develops. Beliefs, values, cultural influences and spiritual needs must be acknowledged. In each case, the patient's needs and circumstances will be recognised.

Flexibility in the CNS–patient relationship is paramount and will vary on a daily basis, and according to the individual patient's needs. In a successful relationship with a patient, the CNS is in a unique position of supportive care provision.

The CNS is also critical in recognising whether support is required for partners, family members or carers and ensuring that it is provided. Family members may also contact the CNS directly for emotional support and education, and the CNS may have valuable advice and information regarding talking to children about cancer.

At a first meeting, an essential contact number for the CNS and an agreement concerning the next point of contact can be suggested. CNSs normally provide a patient/family with a card containing their contact details, and ongoing contacts can be by telephone as well as through face-to-face meetings, either at the time of a hospital appointment or at specifically arranged appointments. Some CNSs are also involved in arranging and facilitating patient groups, which can be a valuable source of peer support.

The MDT should have close working relationships established with a clinical psychologist/counsellor. The introduction of a counsellor can be initiated if and when appropriate. It is essential that the CNS understands and uses the array of available supportive services to optimise emotional well being. This extends to primary care, with liaison with GPs and other community services.

As treatment progresses, the CNS will provide constant reassessment of the patient's psychological needs, aiming to optimise their emotional well being throughout the oncology pathway.

Working as an advocate for the patient is a key part of the role of the CNS, tailoring care to the individual's needs and working towards empowering them to manage and live with the side effects of treatment and/or illness.

Cancer information

The CNS can begin to prepare the patient for treatment by sharing knowledge concerning the diagnosis and suitable treatment options. This may help allay fear and anxiety. Provision of education about the side effects of different treatment modalities can be tailored to the individual in a reassuring way, and in the context of their ongoing management.

Information surveys demonstrate that patients frequently desire more information about treatment options. In helping them understand their treatment options, the CNS ensures fully informed consent and individualised outcome (e.g. choice of breast reconstruction after mastectomy).

Providing an explanation to patients as to how chemotherapy works and why it results in certain side effects can help them understand and better manage these side effects, thus improving treatment compliance. For example, in the case of a gynaecological cancer patient, issues, which may be quite complex, can include menopausal symptoms, lymphoedema, body image and infertility. The CNS is equipped with the knowledge to address these issues with sensitivity, providing advocacy for the patient in sometimes difficult choices.

Side effect management

Once treatment has started, the CNS has a role in informing patients of treatment effects and is proactive in the recognition and management of those side effects. This proactive approach reduces the risk to patients from diseases or treatments.

The CNS can screen patients for disease risk factors or signs of illness, such as thrombotic events and anaemia, and recognise signs and symptoms of oncological emergencies, including neutropenic sepsis (see Chapter 12). By being able to order investigations such as blood tests and recognising the signs and symptoms of neutropenia, the CNS can initiate early appropriate management.

Side effects that the CNS may be able to provide advice on (depending on the tumour group and specific chemotherapy that a patient is undergoing) include nausea/vomiting, taste changes, sore mouth/mouth ulcers, constipation, diarrhoea, peripheral neuropathy and nail changes.

The CNS may be in a position to help with the psychological impact of physical effects such as hair loss, changes to body image, fatigue, fertility considerations, management of iatrogenic menopause, lymphoedema, venous access and specific venous access devices (see Chapter 5).

During chemotherapy, the CNS will telephone patients to monitor their progress. Closely monitoring patients in this way ensures that any side effects can be quickly managed and that the patients are supported through this difficult part of the cancer journey.

The expertise of the CNS may also provide good time management and cost effectiveness. For example, during radiotherapy, head and neck patients require significant input in terms of symptom management during treatment; CNS-led clinics can assess and treat routine oral issues and other related nutritional aspects with the dietitian, supported by the consultant. This enables the patient to tackle the side effects in a timely way, unrestricted by the availability of the consultant. These nurse-led clinics also lead to saved time within consultant appointments.

Sexual health

The close relationship between the CNS and the patient and the ability to spend time focused on symptoms allow the CNS to explore the sensitive areas of sex and sexuality and the impact of cancer treatment upon them.

The urological CNS will support and inform men experiencing erectile dysfunction associated with treatment of prostate cancer or the young man affected by orchidectomy after testicular cancer. The gynaecology CNS may counsel and instruct on the use of vaginal dilators to relieve vaginal stenosis caused by pelvic radiotherapy. The breast CNS may encourage discussion about the vaginal dryness caused by endocrine treatments or the impact on sexuality of changes to body image.

Social and financial considerations

Cancer can have an enormous impact on the finances of a patient and their family. A Macmillan study conducted in Wales demonstrated the average patient losing 20% of employment earnings in the first year after diagnosis and facing costs of treatment (mainly in travel costs) of nearly £400 over 5 years. These costs can be a major stress of treatment and the CNS can provide appropriate links to benefits advice and how to access charitable funding. It is important for the CNS to be proactive in this regard; the Welsh study showed that only one in four patients would discuss these financial issues with a health care professional.

Team liaison and advocacy

The cancer patient is at the centre of a complex medical model involving primary, secondary and tertiary medical care from doctors, nurses and other associated health professionals. The care may take place in different settings and with a variety of teams, sometimes across private and public systems. This can be perplexing for the patient and their carers, and the key worker can help navigate these teams and maintain the appropriate flow of information. With the CNS able to oversee a variety of communications, the patient is more informed and supported, and may preserve a sense of continuity of care. The nurse's knowledge of this wider team and specialisations allows referrals to be made where appropriate, providing a patient-centred, holistic approach.

The CNS can also liaise on the patient's behalf with the consultant at any time with further questions or to discuss options or treatment adjustments that might aid or optimise the patient's emotional and physical well being. This may allow fast-tracking of important problems.

Nurses also facilitate liaison with other health care professionals; for example, a patient developing hypertension on the drug bevacizumab may rely on a cancer nurse within the chemotherapy unit to liaise with primary care to organise appropriate treatment.

The reassuring presence of a familiar CNS may therefore reduce anxiety levels for the patient. If needed, the CNS can be present at appointments with the consultant and in other clinics or settings. In making the transition from one care setting to another (e.g. from surgery to radiotherapy), the CNS preserves continuity of care and can reduce feelings of vulnerability.

Follow up

Many treatment side effects will take long periods to improve and resolve. Patients often report feeling isolated at the end of treatment,

when they are outside the 'safety net' of regular appointments. The relationship between patient and CNS continues beyond the end of the active treatment period.

During this time, the CNS can provide support in promoting survivorship, advice on developing a suitable return-to-work programme and re-evaluation of the patient's work/life balance. By maintaining an open, supportive relationship with the patient, the CNS can also help to build their confidence in looking towards the future.

In the follow-up period, the CNS may continue to advise either in person or over the phone and to liaise as appropriate with the MDT. This mechanism is more convenient and cost effective for the patient, ensures good continuity of care and (in breast cancer) is proven to be safe. As the long-term follow up of cancer is moved into patient-initiated programmes outside secondary or tertiary care (see Chapter 17), the CNS role becomes crucial as a reliable point of referral for the patient seeking advice.

Support outside hospital

Patients may seek and require support in the community. CNSs can provide support and symptom control advice in the patient's home. The majority of these nurses will be specialists in palliative care and will coordinate care for patients who are no longer radically treatable. This care can continue at home or in a hospice environment.

There are several sources for patients seeking support and information outside hospital. The cancer charities Macmillan and Breakthrough Breast Cancer both have telephone helplines staffed by nurses with cancer expertise. Some private medical insurance companies offer a similar service to their members.

There are other examples of charitable sources of support for the cancer patient. Within the UK there are 14 Maggie's Cancer Caring Centres established to provide help for anyone affected by cancer at any point in the cancer journey. These centres are uniquely designed and commissioned from leading architects to provide a welcome refuge from the hospital environment (see Figure 16.2).

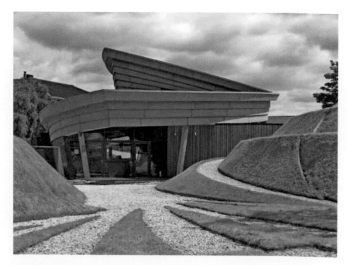

Figure 16.2 The Maggie's Centres are each uniquely designed buildings, built with the purpose of providing a welcoming and supportive space for those affected by cancer.

They run sessions on financial advice and stress management, and help guide patients to the cancer information they need.

There are a large number of specialised volunteer and charitable groups providing support that is specific to a locality, disease site, age group or clinical problem. An online directory of these support groups within the UK is maintained by Macmillan.

Further reading

Fallon, M. & Hanks, G. (eds) (2006) *The ABC of Palliative Care*, 2nd edn. BMJ Books.

Macmillan Cancer Support (2012) Calculating the cost of cancer, http://www.macmillan.org.uk/Documents/GetInvolved/Campaigns/Costofcancer/TheCostofCancercampaignreport.pdf (last accessed 8 March 2013).

Macmillan Cancer Support Web site, www.macmillan.org.uk.

Maggie's Cancer Caring Centre Web site, www.maggiescentres.org.

National Cancer Action Team (2010) Quality in nursing: clinical nurse specialists in cancer care – provision, proportion and performance, http://ncat.nhs.uk/sites/default/files/Census%20of%20CNS%20Workforce%202010.pdf (last accessed 8 March 2013).

Royal College of Nurses (2005) Maxi nurses: nurses working in advanced and extended roles promoting and developing patient-centred health care, http://www.rcn.org.uk/__data/assets/pdf_file/0004/78646/002511.pdf (last accessed 8 March 2013).

CHAPTER 17

Cancer Survivorship

Esther Bird[1], Amy Guppy[2], and Carlo Palmieri[3]

[1]Silverdale GP Surgery, Burgess Hill, West Sussex, UK
[2]Mount Vernon Cancer Centre and Hillingdon Hospitals NHS Foundation Trust, Northwood, Herts, UK
[3]University of Liverpool, Department of Molecular and Clinical Cancer Medicine, The Royal Liverpool University Hospital & The Clatterbridge Cancer Centre, Liverpool, UK

OVERVIEW

- An estimated 2 million living people in the UK have a cancer history, with estimates of 4 million survivors by 2030
- 50% are breast, prostate and colorectal cancer patients
- 50% of adults survive more than 5 years
- There is a 3.2% growth per year in number of survivors
- Many cancer survivors live with the long-term sequelae of their treatment and negative impact on their quality of life. In addition, cancer treatments are associated with toxicities that impact on long-term health

---

Cancer survival

Improvements in care have led to steady improvement in long-term cancer survival, with average survival at 10 years today being 46%, compared with 23% 30 years ago. The 5-year survival rate is now approaching 50% of all patients. With high levels of cancer incidence (see Table 17.1), survivorship has become a major issue.

Morbidity secondary to cancer treatment

Improvements in outcomes have led to the problem of how best to manage the long-term toxicities of treatment. Some effects are common, some much less so (see Box 17.1). They can develop months to years after treatment and range from cardiovascular and cognitive issues to risks of secondary malignancies. Specialist

---

Box 17.1 **Consequence of cancer treatment related to incidence**

- *Rare consequences*: e.g. radiation-induced brachial plexopathy following radiotherapy for breast cancer.
- *Less common consequences*: e.g. chronic gastrointestinal syndromes following pelvic radiotherapy.
- *Common consequences*: e.g. osteoporosis, and sexual dysfunction.

ABC of Cancer Care, First Edition.
Edited by Carlo Palmieri, Esther Bird and Richard Simcock.
© 2013 John Wiley & Sons, Ltd. Published 2013 by John Wiley & Sons, Ltd.

Table 17.1 Cancer prevalence in the UK in 2008. Reprinted by permission from Macmillan Publishers Ltd on behalf of Cancer Research UK: Maddams J, Brewster D, Gavin A, Steward J, Elliott J, Utley M & Møller H, Cancer prevalence in the United Kingdom: estimates for 2008. BrJ Cancer (2009) 101:541–547.

	UK	%
Total	2 002 516	100.0
By sex		
Male	819 188	40.9
Female	1 183 328	59.1
By age		
0–17	15 073	0.8
18–64	729 181	36.4
65+	1 258 262	62.8
By cancer type		
Breast	548 998	27.4
Colorectal	235 816	11.8
Prostate	253 436	12.7
Lung	63 522	3.2
Other	900 744	45.0

follow up is usually only for a limited period, typically 3–5 years, and therefore primary care will have an increasing role in caring for cancer survivors. Education, information and resources to enable recognition and effective management of relevant issues are vital.

Chronic effects of cancer treatment

Surviving cancer does not guarantee good health. A 2008 Macmillan survey found that 90% of cancer survivors had visited their GP in the previous 12 months, compared to 68% of the wider population. Even 10 years after diagnosis, breast and colorectal patients are more likely to visit their GP. Many organ systems may be affected (see Table 17.2). A matched cohort analysis of longitudinal primary care records from over 26 000 cancer survivors demonstrated an increased risk of osteoporosis, heart failure, coronary artery disease and hypothyroidism: chronic illnesses directly related to cancer treatments. Additionally, there may be psychological and social consequences to cancer treatment.

Gastrointestinal problems

Chronic gastrointestinal (GI) problems following cancer treatment can affect any part of the GI tract. Pelvic radiotherapy is particularly

Table 17.2 Organ-specific consequences of cancer treatment.

Organ system	Late effects/sequelae of radiotherapy	Late effects/sequelae of chemotherapy	Examples of cytotoxic drugs responsible
Bones/soft tissues	Short stature Osteonecrosis	Avascular necrosis	Steroids
Heart	Coronary artery disease Pericarditis Pericardial effusion	Cardiomyopathy Heart failure	Anthracyclines Cyclophosphamides Trastuzumab
Lungs	Pulmonary fibrosis	Pulmonary fibrosis	Bleomycin Carmustine (BCNU)
Central nervous system	Neuropsychological impairment	Neuropsychological impairment	Methotrexate
Peripheral nervous system		Peripheral neuropathy	Taxanes Platinum-containing agents Vinca alkaloids
Blood	Cytopenia Myelodysplasia	Myelodysplastic syndromes	Alkylating agents
Kidney	Renal impairment	Renal impairment	Cisplatin
Gut	Malabsorption Stricture	Hepatic fibrosis Cirrhosis	Methotrexate Carmustine
Genitourinary	Bladder fibrosis	Bladder fibrosis Haemorrhagic cystitis	Cyclophosphamide
Gonadal	Sterility Premature menopause	Sterility Premature menopause	Alkylating agents
Pituitary	Primary pituitary failure Growth hormone deficiency		
Thyroid	Hypothyroidism Thyroid nodules		
Eyes	Cataracts Retinopathy	Cataracts	Steroids

associated with bowel issues, as well as affecting bladder and sexual function (see Chapter 8). The number of cases of pelvic irradiation illness is comparable with the number of new cases of inflammatory bowel disease (approximately 8000/annum), but most hospitals only have a service for the latter. The British Society of Gastroenterologists published guidance on managing chronic GI problems following cancer treatment, and importantly on who should be referred for specialist input; this is a useful and timely resource for those caring for such patients.

Bone health

Cancer survivors have a higher incidence of osteoporosis than the general population. Chemotherapy-induced menopause, gonadotrophin-releasing hormone (GnRH) suppression of gonadal function, aromatase inhibitors (see Chapter 9) and glucocorticoids all accelerate bone loss and can impact negatively on bone health long-term. Prostate and breast cancer survivors are at particular risk of accelerated bone loss and osteoporosis as a result of endocrine therapy. Patients at risk of bone loss secondary to their cancer treatment should be assessed for possible causes of secondary osteoporosis and osteoporotic fracture, and these should be managed accordingly.

Dual-energy x-ray absorptiometry (DEXA) is used to asses bone mineral density, and in postmenopausal women and men over 50 years of age the T-score is the relevant measure for assessing bone

health. According to World Health Organization (WHO) criteria, osteoporosis is a bone mineral density 2.5 standard deviations or more below the average value for a young healthy adult of the same sex (a T-score of <2.5 standard deviations). The WHO Fracture Assessment Tool (FRAX) (http://www.shef.ac.uk/FRAX) can be used as a clinical aid to assess an individual's osteoporotic fracture risk, with or without bone mineral density measurements. All cancer patients at risk of bone loss should have a baseline DEXA and be managed appropriately based on the result. This may include lifestyle advice (such as weight-bearing exercise (e.g. walking), avoidance of smoking, moderation of alcohol intake and sensible exposure to sunlight), the use of vitamin D and calcium (≥ 1 g calcium and ≥ 800 IU vitamin D) or pharmacological treatments approved for osteoporosis, such as bisphosphonates and the receptor activator of nuclear factor-kB (RANK) ligand inhibitor, denusomab. Figure 17.1 outlines a general algorithm for patients at risk of cancer treatment-related bone loss.

Sexual dysfunction

In a survey of over 1000 cancer patients who had completed treatment, changes in sexual interest were reported in 42% of prostate and 20% of breast survivors. Erectile dysfunction was reported in 46% of prostate and 31% of colorectal patients. These findings have been replicated in a prospective study of over 26 000 breast, colorectal and prostate patients matched to noncancer controls.

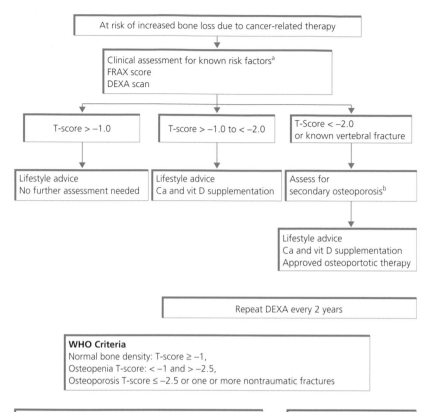

At risk of increased bone loss due to cancer-related therapy

Clinical assessment for known risk factors[a]
FRAX score
DEXA scan

T-score > −1.0

T-score > −1.0 to < −2.0

T-Score < −2.0
or known vertebral fracture

Lifestyle advice
No further assessment needed

Lifestyle advice
Ca and vit D supplementation

Assess for
secondary osteoporosis[b]

Lifestyle advice
Ca and vit D supplementation
Approved osteoportotic therapy

Repeat DEXA every 2 years

WHO Criteria
Normal bone density: T-score ≥ −1,
Osteopenia T-score: < −1 and > −2.5,
Osteoporosis T-score ≤ −2.5 or one or more nontraumatic fractures

[a]**Risk Factors for Osteoporotic Fracture**
Previous fragility fracture above the age of 50 years
Parental history of fracture
A body mass index (BMI) of <22
Alcohol consumption > 4 units per day
Prior oral corticosteroid use for more than 6 months
Diseases associated with secondary osteoporosis

[b]**Suggested Assessment**
ESR
FBC
Liver function test
Ca^{2+}, phosphate
Serum creatinine
Endomysial antibody
Serum TSH

Figure 17.1 General algorithm for assessing and managing bone health in cancer patients at risk of cancer treatment-related bone loss. ESR, erythocyte sedimentation rate; FBC, full blood count; TSH, thyroid stimulating hormone.

Sexual dysfunction can result from both physical and psychological issues. These include alterations in body image, anxiety, depression and physical issues such as vaginal atrophy and erectile dysfunction. Physical causes can be due to pelvic/perineal surgery or potential nerve damage (seen with radical prostatectomy or lymph node dissection in testicular cancer). Chemotherapy can result in premature gonadal failure, and endocrine therapy can result in lowered circulating sex hormones. Radiotherapy to the pelvis can result in vaginal fibrosis (see Chapter 8).

Hormone replacement therapy (HRT) is an option in women with early ovarian failure (although contraindicated after some breast cancers) and men with premature testicular failure. Potential interventions for erectile dysfunction include phosphodiesterase inhibitors such as sildenafil, intraurethral suppository or intracavernosal alprostadil, venous and vacuum constriction devices and penile prosthesis implants. Referral to menopause clinics for problematic menopausal symptoms can be considered, as can referral for psychosexual counselling, depending on the underlying issues.

Fertility issues

Fertility may be compromised by effects of treatment on sexual or gonadal function. Whenever possible, measures to preserve fertility should be taken prior to commencing definitive treatment (e.g. sperm storage or *in vitro* fertility treatment). Post-treatment, natural conception should be tried, but if unsuccessful then referral to a fertility unit is required. Adoption is an option for cancer survivors but the process requires a medical report from an oncologist regarding both history and prognosis.

Cardiovascular disease

Ischaemic heart disease and heart failure are potential toxicities of cancer treatment. Mediastinal and left-sided breast radiotherapy can result in incidental irradiation of the heart and lead to radiation-induced coronary artery disease. Improved radiotherapy techniques minimise cardiac dose. The anthracyclines (epirubicin and doxorubicin) are an important class of cytotoxic but are known to cause heart failure long-term. Women with breast cancer treated with anthracycline-based chemotherapy had a 50% higher cardiac mortality compared to those exposed to a non-anthracycline regimen. After testicular cancer there is increased risk of cardiovascular disease, caused by an increased incidence of metabolic syndrome (hypertension, dyslipidemia, obesity and insulin resistance), which has been linked to cisplatin chemotherapy and hypogonadism.

Patients exposed to cancer treatments associated with increased cardiovascular risk should be assessed, given lifestyle advice and have modifiable risk factors (e.g. hypertension and dyslipidemia) appropriately managed.

Secondary malignancies

Secondary malignancies may arise due to genetic syndromes or be related to the previous cancer treatment. Chemotherapy, radiotherapy and tamoxifen are associated with secondary malignancies. Leukaemia as a secondary cancer can occur following treatment with chemotherapy, in particular with alkylating agents. Secondary malignancies in survivors of haematological cancers are well described, with a standardised incidence ratio (SIR) of 6.3 and 4.6 in leukaemia and lymphoma patients, respectively. Younger patients are at higher risk of developing a later cancer, with patients diagnosed at 10 years or less at higher risk than adult patients (SIR 10.6 versus 4.0).

Cancers may develop in an irradiated area. Women treated with radiotherapy for Hodgkin's disease before the age of 30 have a 12–25-fold increased risk of breast cancer. These women should have annual breast screening with magnetic resonance imaging (MRI) until the age of 50. Thyroid cancer is the most common post-radiation cancer noted in Hodgkin's disease survivors. Tamoxifen (widely used in breast cancer) is associated with endometrial cancer.

Knowledge of the risk of secondary malignancies, particularly in the paediatric setting, has led to treatment modifications. Patients should be counselled about risk and given advice about risk-reducing lifestyle modification and possible symptoms that should lead them to seek medical advice, particularly as they may occur years after treatment.

Psychological issues

Acute grief reactions, anxiety and panic attacks, increased suicidal tendency and thoughts of euthanasia can all manifest more commonly after a cancer diagnosis. Reduced self-confidence can be a barrier to accessing support. Routinely asking patients about mental health symptoms using open questions and validated screening tools is vital. Holistic services in the hospital and community that focus not just on treatment and outcomes but also on mood and easing life adjustments make valuable contributions. Clinical nurse specialists (see Chapter 16) are instrumental to the quality of care received by patients.

Employment and finance

The social and economic dimensions of cancer should not be underestimated.

There are currently more than 700 000 people of working age in the UK with a cancer diagnosis. Patients face a drop in income, especially if self-employed, from the need to take time off for treatment and recovery, in some cases permanently. Treatment incurs increased costs, such as travel to hospitals and special dietary requirements. Cancer survivors may face problems on returning to work, such as fatigue and neuropathy. Not all employers have occupational health provision and a phased return to work may be hard to manage. Patients may face discrimination in the workplace despite its being illegal. Many organisations (e.g. Macmillan and Maggie's Cancer Caring Centre) provide support to patients with regard to benefits, returning to work and legal rights. Health care professionals should signpost places to receive help and provide information on the impact of treatment on work.

Unmet need

Cancer patients and survivors have significant unmet care and support needs. At the end of treatment, 30% of patients have five or more moderate or severe unmet needs, many persisting for months. Inadequate education regarding the symptoms and signs of relapse, fear of recurrence, depression reducing self-confidence, sexual issues and financial shortfalls can be some of the difficulties experienced.

Surveys of cancer survivors have highlighted failure to provide personalised information regarding cancer treatment, risk of recurrence and potential long-term consequences of treatment.

Survivorship initiatives

The National Cancer Survivorship Initiative (NCSI) was set up as a recommendation in the Cancer Reform Strategy (Department of Health 2007), and its work was reinforced in Improving Outcomes: A Strategy for Cancer (Department of Health 2011). The NCSI vision states that cancer survivors should be supported to live as healthy and active a life as is possible for as long as possible, with models of aftercare focussing on supported self-management and addressing known unmet needs.

Traditionally, cancer patients' follow up has been based on a medical (illness) model, where patients are seen regularly in a hospital-based outpatient environment for up to 5 years. Regular follow-up visits entail a financial and emotional cost for the patient, and the model fails to address the survivor's needs. Furthermore, rising incidence and survival rates make the traditional model unsustainable from a resource perspective.

The NCSI has piloted a supported self-managed follow-up model of care for breast, prostate, lung and colorectal cancer survivors, aimed at meeting key needs (see Box 17.2). In this model, patients receive a holistic needs assessment on completion of treatment, giving them the opportunity to discuss concerns and fears and allowing time to signpost appropriate services. Patients receive personalised care plans and treatment summaries, as well as detailed information regarding signs and symptoms of disease recurrence and point-of-contact information by which to reaccess the system if necessary. Remote monitoring systems, such as mammography, regular tumour marker tests and colonoscopy, are used to ensure that patients are called promptly for surveillance tests in the community, without the need for a clinic visit. Initial findings suggest that this model of care is both safe and acceptable to cancer survivors. Personalised information empowers both the patient and their GP to recognise symptoms of recurrence and potential late toxicity.

Survivorship courses

The end of cancer treatment may be a 'teachable moment': a point at which lifestyle changes can be discussed and potentially modified. Patient education and wider access to community-based programmes will facilitate this.

A number of mentoring courses are now available to help patients with the transition from treatment to follow up. 'Where Now?' (run by Maggies's Cancer Caring Centres) aims to provide patients with the tools to deal with the issues that they may face on completing cancer treatment. Patients are also given information and taught skills to optimise their health in terms of exercise, nutrition and emotional and medical issues.

Exercise

Exercise can prevent and manage some of the problems associated with cancer and cancer treatment, including depression and fatigue.

Exercise after cancer should be encouraged. Published data show exercise to be safe, although the nature, duration and intensity of any such exercise should be tailored to the individual. A meta-analysis of published controlled intervention studies has shown significant small to moderate improvements in aerobic fitness, body weight and body fat, quality of life and fatigue for patients who exercise.

Obesity is established as a risk factor for a number of cancers. In addition, it is a poor prognostic factor among survivors of breast and colon cancers. Given this and other known obesity health issues such as diabetes and cardiovascular disease, increased exercise and dietary modifications (see Chapter 14) should be recommended to breast and colon cancer survivors.

Further reading

British Association of Sport and Exercise Sciences (2011) The BASES expert statement on exercise and cancer survivorship. *Sport and Exercise Scientist*, **28**, 16–17.

Department of Health (2007) Cancer Reform Strategy, http://www.dh.gov.uk/en/Publicationsandstatistics/Publications/PublicationsPolicyAndGuidance/DH_081006 (last accessed 8 March 2013).

Department of Health (2010) The National Cancer Survivorship Initiative vision, http://www.ncsi.org.uk/wp-content/uploads/NCSI-Vision-Document.pdf (last accessed 8 March 2013).

Department of Health (2011) Improving Outcomes: a Strategy for Cancer, http://www.dh.gov.uk/en/Publicationsandstatistics/Publications/PublicationsPolicyAndGuidance/DH_123371 (last accessed 8 March 2013).

Andreyev, H.J.N., Davidson, S., Gillespie, C., Allum, W.H. & Swarbrick, E. (2012) Practice guidance on the management of acute and chronic gastrointestinal problems arising as a result of treatment for cancer. *Gut*, **61**, 179–192.

Lustberg, M.B., Reinbolt, R.E. & Shapiro, C.L. (2012) Bone health in adult cancer survivorship. *Journal of Clinical Oncology*, **30**, 3665–3674.

Macmillan Cancer Support (2011) The importance of physical activity for people living with and beyond cancer: a concise evidence review, http://www.macmillan.org.uk/Documents/AboutUs/Commissioners/Physicalactivityevidencereview.pdf (last accessed 8 March 2013).

Macmillan Cancer Support Web site, www.macmillan.org.uk.

Maggie's Cancer Caring Centre Web site, www.maggiescentres.org.

Maddams, J., Brewster, D., Gavin, A., Steward, J., Elliott, J., Utley, M. & Møller, H. (2009) Cancer prevalence in the United Kingdom: estimates for 2008. *British Journal of Cancer*, **101**, 541–547.

National Cancer Survivorship Initiative Web site, www.ncsi.org.uk.

Reid, D.M., Doughty, J., Eastell, R., Heys, S.D., Howell, A., McCloskey, E.V. et al. (2008) Guidance for the management of breast cancer treatment-induced bone loss: a consensus position statement from a UK expert group. *Cancer Treatment Review*, **34**, S1–S18.

Richards, M., Corner, J. & Maher, J. (2011) The National Cancer Survivorship Initiative: new and emerging evidence on the ongoing needs of cancer survivors. *British Journal of Cancer*, **105**, S1–S4.

Woodward, E., Jessop, M., Glaser, A., Stark, D. (2011) Late effects in survivors of teenage and young adult cancer: does age matter? *Ann Oncol*, **22**, 2561–8.

Index

abdominoperineal resection of the rectum
(APR), 14
abiraterone, 40, 42
ablation techniques, 19
acetyl groups, 46
acupuncture, 70
adjuvant therapy, 3
chemotherapy, 21
endocrine therapy, 40
radiotherapy, 35
tamoxifen therapy, 40
adrenocorticotropic hormone (ACTH), 42
Advisory Committee on Borderline Substances
(ACBS), 66
ageing population and cancer, 61
ageing process and changes, 61–62
effects on pharmacokinetics, 62
interindividual variation in function, 62
nutritional status, 62
social and neuropsychological changes, 62
alemtuzumab, 46
alginate dressings, 34
algorithm of patient pathways for lung and
colorectal cancer, 9
alitretinoin, 46
alkylating agents, 23
alopecia
chemotherapy-induced, 26
radiation-induced, 35
American Joint Committee on Cancer (AJCC), 3
amikacin, 56
anastomosis, 14
anastrozole, 40
anemia, chemotherapy-induced, 26–27
angiotensin-converting enzyme (ACE)
inhibitors, 29
anthracyclines, 23, 80
antidiarrhoea medications, 25
antiemetics, 25, 28
antigen-presenting cells (APCs), 47
Ara-C, 27
aromatase inhibitors, 39–42
aromatherapy, 72
autologous reconstruction techniques, 13
autonomic neuropathy, 28
axillary clearance, 11
axillary metastatic disease in breast cancer, 11

benzodiazepines, 59
beta blockers, 29

bevacizumab, 46
bexarotene, 46
bicalutamide, 42, 43
biological therapy
monoclonal antibodies (mABs), 45–46
tyrosine kinases, 44–45
biomarkers, 52–54
approaches to detection of, 53
clinical utilities, 52
defined, 52
historical perspective, 53
modern, 52
bladder cancer, 29
bleeding, 27
bleomycin, 24, 28
bone loss, 79
bone marrow suppression, radiation-induced, 35
bone metastases
bone scintigraphic evaluation, 16
fixation of long bones, 16
from renal cell carcinoma (RCC), 16
bone scanning, 9
bortezomib, 45
brachytherapy, 32, 42
B-RAF, 44
brain metastases, 18
breast cancer, 32, 82
axillary metastatic disease in, 11
male, 41
sentinel lymph node biopsy (SLNB) in, 11
breast care nurse, 11
breast conserving surgery (BCS), 10, 12
breast irradiation, 36
breast reconstruction, 13

CA125, 53
calcitonin, 58
Calman–Hine report, 1
Cancer Act, 1939, 73
cancer care, 1
Cancer Networks, 1, 22
cancer survivors, 82
cancer treatment, chronic effects of, 78–79
cancer waiting times, 2–3
capecitabine, 23, 24
capsular contracture, 13
capsulotomy/capsulectomy, 13
carboplatin, 23, 24, 28, 59
cardiac toxicity of chemotherapy, 26, 28–29
cardiomyopathy, chemotherapy-induced, 29
cardiovascular disease, 80–81

ceftazidime, 56
cellulitis, 22
central nervous system (CNS), 19
central venous access device (CVAD), 22
cetuximab, 33, 46, 59
chemoreceptor trigger zone, 28
chemotherapy, 10, 44, 57, 80, 81
administration of, 22
chemotherapeutic agents, 24
CVAD devices for, 23
cytotoxic effects, 23
dosing and schedule, 23–25
effect on nutritional status, 64–65
intravenous (IV), 20, 22
modes of action of, 23–25
NHS cancer strategies and, 21–22
oral administration, 22
treatment settings, 20–21
chest x-ray (CXR), 5, 28, 59
Chinese and herbal medicines, 72
chiropractic, 71
chronic myeloid leukaemia (CML), 44
chronic obstructive pulmonary disease
(COPD), 27
cisplatin, 24, 28, 29, 59
cladribine, 24
clinical nurse specialists (CNSs)
CNS–patient relationship, 75
cost-related advice to patients, 76
emotional support to patients, role in
offering, 74–76, 74–77
follow-up with patients, 76
led clinics, 75
side effects management, 75
team liaison and advocacy, 76
clinical trials
biomarkers in, 52–54
categories of, 50
defined, 50
drug development process, 50–51
in elderly population, 61
ethical principles, 52
phases of, 51–52
trial design, 52
Cobalt[60], 30
colony stimulating factors (CSFs), 49
Common Toxicity Criteria (CTC), 26
complementary and alternative medicines
(CAMs)
acupuncture, 70

complementary and alternative medicines (CAMs)
(*continued*)
advice to, 73
aromatherapy, 72
background, 69
Chinese and herbal medicines, 72
chiropractic, 71
evidence for, 70
grouping of, 70
homeopathy, 72
massage and manipulation techniques, 71
patient safety and, 73
reasons for choosing, 69
Reiki, 73
sources of information, 73
spirituality, 72–73
Comprehensive Geriatric Assessment (CGA), 63
computed tomography (CT), 5–9, 28, 30
plan of prostate radiotherapy, 31
of spinal metastases, 16–17
SVCO, 57
computer-assisted surgery (CAS), 12
corticosteroids, 58, 59
cosmesis, 13
crizotinib, 45
cryotherapy, 19
Cybernife, 18, 33
cyclophosphamide, 24, 29
cytochrome P450(17)alpha (CYP17), 42

dacarbazine, 24
dactinomycin, 24
dasatanib, 45
daunorubicin, 24
da Vinci system, 12–13
deep inferior epigastric perforator flap (DIEP), 13
denusomab, 79
dexamethasone, 17, 36, 59
diarrhoea, 59, 67
chemotherapy-induced, 26, 27
radiation-induced, 37
digital mammography, 5–6
docetaxel, 24, 28, 43
doxorubicin, 24, 28, 80
drug development process, 50–51
drug limiting toxicity (DLT), 51
dry mouth (Xerostomia), 67
dual-energy x-ray absorptiometry (DXA),
41, 79
ductal carcinoma in situ (DCIS), 6
dysphagia, 67

Early Breast Cancer Trialists' Collaborative Group
(EBCTC), 40
ECOG/WHO/ZUBUD performance status
score, 4
effective multidisciplinary team (MDT), 3–4
elderly, cancer in, 61
challenges in managing, 61–63
Comprehensive Geriatric Assessment
(CGA), 63
optimising care, 63
emergency radiotherapy, 32
of spinal cord compression, 32
of superior vena cava obstruction (SVCO), 32
emergency surgery in oncology, 14. *see also*
oncology emergencies

ENCODE, 49
endocrine therapy
adjuvant, 40
combination with targeted therapy, 41
current, 39–40
in neoadjuvant setting, 41
postmenopausal women, 40
premenopausal women, 40–41
in prostate cancer, 42–43
side effects of, 40–42
toxicity, 43
endoscopic mastectomy, 12
endoscopic ultrasound (EUS), 6
'enhanced recovery programmes' (ERPs),
11, 64
enteral tube feeding, 68
enzalutamide, 40, 42
ephedrine hydrochloride, 37
epirubicin, 24, 28, 80
erectile dysfunction, 80
erlotinib (Tarceva), 45
European Organisation for Research and
Treatment of Cancer (EORTC), 26
exemestane, 40–41
everolimus, 45
exercise, 82
extended neck dissection, 12
extravasation, 22

febrile neutropenia, 55
fertility issues, 80
^{18}F-FDG PET-CT, 9
fludarabine, 24
fluoroscopy, 5
5-fluorouracil, 24
follicle stimulating hormone (FSH), 39
Fracture Assessment Tool (FRAX), 79
fulvestrant, 39–40
functional MRI, 18

gallium, 58
Gama Knife, 18
gastrointestinal (GI) problems, 79
toxicities of radiotherapy, 37
gastrointestinal (GI) resections, 11, 14
gefitinib, 45
gemcitabine, 24
General Regulatory Council for Complementary
Therapies (GRCCT), 70
Genome Project, 49
genomics, 53
gentamicin, 56
germinal epithelium, 29
GI toxicity of chemotherapy, 27
gonadal ablation, 41
gonadotrophin releasing hormone (GnRH), 39
analogues, 29
Good Clinical Practice (GCP), 52
goserelin, 29, 42
granulocyte colony stimulating factors
(GCSFs), 23, 25, 27, 49, 56
Groshong lines, 23
groupthink, 2

haematological toxicity of chemotherapy, 27
haemorrhoids, 38
hair loss, chemotherapy-induced, 26

Helsinki Declaration, 1964, 52
HER-1, 46
HER-2, 44, 46, 49
Hickman lines, 23
high-dose-rate (HDR) brachytherapy, 32
histone deacetylases (HDACs), 46
Hodgkin lymphoma, 29, 81
homeopathy, 72
hormone replacement therapy (HRT), 80
5HT$_3$ antagonists, 28
hydrocolloid, 34
hydrocortisone, 34
hypercalcaemia, malignant, 57–58
management, 58
pathophysiology, 58
treatment, 58
hypomagnasaemia, 59

ifosphamide, 24
image-guided radiotherapy, 32
imaging tests in oncology, 5–9
imatinib, 44, 45
immediate breast reconstruction (IMBR), 13
implants, 13
independent data monitoring committee
(IDMC), 52
inferior gluteal artery perforator/'iGAP' flap,
14
intensity-modulated radiotherapy, 32
intent of treatment, 2–3
interferon, 46–47
interferon alpha (Roferon, Intron A), 47
interleukin-2 (Aldesleukin®), 47
interleukin (immunotherapy), 46–47
International Registry of Lung Metastases, 19
intraoperative radiotherapy, 32
intraperitoneal chemotherapy, 23
intrathecal chemotherapy, 23
intravenous (IV) chemotherapy, 20
in vitro fertilisation (IVF), 29
ipilimumab, 46
irinotecan, 27

Karnofsky Performance Status score, 3
ketaconzole, 42
kyphoplasty, 18

β-lactam agent, 56
laparoscopy, 12
lapatinib (Tyverb), 44, 45
laser interstitial thermal therapy (LITT), 19
latissimus dorsi (LD) pedicled flap, 13
letrozole, 41
leuprolin, 42
linear accelerator (LinAc), 30, 32
liver anatomy, Couinaud classification, 19
liver (hepatic) metastases, 18–19
liver resection, 19
lorazepam, 59
lung injury, chemotherapy-induced, 28
lung metastases, 19
luteinising hormone (LH), 39
lymphangitis carcinomatosis, 58–59
lymphoedema, 37

mAB ipilimumab (YERVOY), 46
macrometastases, defined, 15

magnetic resonance imaging (MRI), 7–9, 30
   functional, 18
   whole-spine, 16
male breast cancer, 41
malignant hypercalcaemia, 57–58
mammography, 5–6
Manual for Cancer Services, 1
margin related to oncological resection, 12–13
massage and manipulation techniques, 71
mastectomy, 12
maximum tolerated dose (MTD), 51
Melonin, 34
melphalan, 24
Mepilex, 34
6-mercaptopurine, 24
meropenem, 56
metabolomics, 53
metastasis
   bone, 16
   brain, 18
   liver, 18–19
   lung, 19
   macrometastases, defined, 15
   micrometastases, defined, 15
   oligometastatic disease, 15
   sites of, 15
   spine, 16–18
metastatic/advanced disease, 40–42
metastatic spinal cord compression (MSCC), 16, 56–57
methicillin-resistant *Staphylococcus aureus* (MRSA), 5
methotrexate, 24
methylphenidate, 35
metoclopramide, 28
microbubbles, 6
microcalcification (MCC), detection of, 5
micrometastases, defined, 15
Mirels scoring system, 16
modified radical neck dissection, 12
motor neuropathy, 28
6MP, 27
mucositis, 35–36
multidisciplinary team (MDT), 74
   for breast and head and neck cancer, 2
   databases of, 2
   defined, 1
   effective, 3–4
   membership of, 1
   Network specialist MDT, 1
multidisciplinary team meeting (MDTM), 1
multileaf collimators, 30
Multinational Association for Supportive Care in Cancer (MASCC) scoring index, 56
myelography, 17
myelosuppression, 27

National Cancer Action Team (NCAT), 1, 2, 22
National Cancer Survivorship Initiative (NCSI), 81
National Confidential Enquiry into Patient Outcome and Death (NCEPOD) report, 22
National Institute for Health and Clinical Excellence (NICE), 12, 72
National Lung Screening Trial (NLST), 7
nausea, 26, 28, 67
neoadjuvant therapy, 21

network specialist MDT, 1
neurological toxicity of chemotherapy, 28
neutropenia, 26, 27
neutropenic sepsis, 55–56
nilotinib, 45
non-Hodgkin lymphoma, 29
nonsteroidal anti-inflammatory drugs (NSAIDs), 22
nuclear medicine studies, 8–9
nurse. *see also* clinical nurse specialists (CNSs)
   breast care, 11
   stoma, 11
nutritional status
   chemotherapy and biological agents, effect of, 64–65
   depletion and malnutrition in cancer patient, 64
   enteral tube feeding, 68
   goals of nutrition intervention, 65
   oral nutritional supplements (ONS), 66–68
   parenteral nutrition, role of, 68
   radiotherapy, effect of, 65–66
   surgery implications on, 64
   vitamins and minerals, 68
   weight control and exercise, 68
nutrition impact symptoms, 65

oesophageal ulceration, 36
oestrogen receptor (ER) positive breast cancer, 39
ofatumumab, 46
oligometastatic disease, 15
oncogene addiction, 49
oncology emergencies
   hypomagnasaemia, 59
   lymphangitis carcinomatosis, 58–59
   malignant hypercalcaemia, 57–58
   metastatic spinal cord compression (MSCC), 56–57
   neutropenic sepsis, 55–56
   superior vena cava obstruction (SVCO), 57
oncoplastic surgery, 13
one-step nucleic acid amplification (OSNA), 12
opioids, 59
oral magnesium therapy, 59
oral nutritional supplements (ONS), 66–68
organ-specific consequences of cancer treatment, 79
orthopaedic fixation for bone disease, 16
ovarian radiation, effect of, 38
oxaliplatin, 24, 28
oxcetocaine, 36

paclitaxel, 24, 28
palliative chemotherapy, 21
panitumumab, 46
paralytic ileus, 28
parenteral nutrition, 68
patey mastectomy, 12
percutaneous ethanol injection (PEI), 19
peripherally inserted central catheter (PICC), 23
peripheral neuropathy, chemotherapy-induced, 26
perspex shells, 31
pertuzumab, 46, 47
phase I clinical trials, 51
phase II clinical trials, 51
phase III clinical trials, 51–52

phase IV clinical trials, 52
photodynamic therapy (PDT), 19
photon radiation, 30
physiological tremor filtration, 12
piperacillin/tazobactam, 56
plain-film radiography, 5
plantar palmar erythema syndrome, 23
platinum compounds, 23
positron emission tomography – computed tomography (PET-CT), 7–9, 33
proctitis, 37
prostatic acid phosphatase (PAP), 47
proteomics, 53
psychological issues, 81
PTH-related peptide (PTRrP), 58
pulmonary metastasectomy, 19
pulmonary toxicity of chemotherapy, 26, 28
pyrimidines, 23

radial forearm free flap (RFFF), 13
radical Halstead mastectomy, 12
radical neck dissection, 12
radical radiotherapy, 32
radical surgery (prostatectomy), 42
radiofrequency ablation (RFA), 19
radiological staging of cancer
   endoscopic ultrasound (EUS), 6
   fluoroscopy, 5
   mammography, 5–6
   plain-film radiography, 5
   TNM staging, 5
   ultrasound, 6
radiosensitivity of different tumour types, 31
radiotherapy, 10, 80
   advanced technologies, 32–33
   doses, 30–31
   effect on nutritional status, 65–66
   emergency, 32
   image-guided, 32
   intensity-modulated, 32
   intraoperative, 32
   investment in, 33
   for MSCC, 17
   oral care during, 35
   palliative treatments, 32
   positioning in, 30
   radical, 32
   radiobiological principles, 31–32
   stereotactic, 32
   treatment practicalities, 30–31
   whole-brain, 18, 35
RANK (receptor activator of nuclear factor-kB) ligand inhibitors, 58
rational drug design, 44
reconstruction surgery in oncology, 13–14
   abdominoperineal resection of the rectum (APR), 14
   anastomosis, 14
   breast, 13
   deep inferior epigastric perforator flap (DIEP), 13
   gastrointestinal (GI) resections, 11, 14
   inferior gluteal artery perforator/'iGAP' flap, 14
   latissimus dorsi (LD), 13
   radial forearm free flap (RFFF), 13
   total mesorectal excision (TME), 14

reconstruction surgery in oncology (*continued*)
transverse abdominis muscle flap
(TRAM), 13
rectal stump, 14
Reiki, 73
renal cell carcinoma (RCC), 16
resection margin, significance of, 12–13
respiratory tract infection (RTI), 28
retinoic acid, 46
rituximab, 46
romidepsin, 46

scalp hypothermia ('cold capping'), 26
sclerosant, 19
secondary malignancies selective internal
radiotherapy, 19, 81
selective neck dissection, 12
sentinel lymph node biopsy (SLNB) in breast
cancer, 11
sexual dysfunction, 79–80
sigmoidoscopy, 38
silver sulfadiazine lyofoam, 34
simple mastectomy, 12
sipuleucel-T (Provenge), 47
skin radiation reactions, 34
skin sparing mastectomy, 12
SIR-Spheres, 19
small-cell lung cancer (SCLC), 57
social and economic dimensions of cancer, 81
sorafenib, 45
sperm banking, 29
spine metastases, 16–18
surgery for, 17–18
staging of cancer, 3
stereotactic radiosurgery (SRS), 18, 32
stoma nurse, 11
subcutaneous implanted venous access, 23
subcutaneous mastectomy, 12
sunitinib, 45
superior vena cava obstruction (SVCO), 57
surgery for patients with metastases
of bone metastases, 16
of brain metastases, 18
of liver (hepatic) metastases, 18–19
of lung metastases, 19
preoperative considerations, 15
surgery in oncology. *see also* emergency
radiotherapy; oncology emergencies
axillary clearance, 11
bowel preparation, 14
breast-conserving, 10, 12
computer-assisted surgery (CAS), 12
'dual localisation' technique, 11
elements and modalities of preoperative
staging, 10
emergency, 14

'enhanced recovery programmes' (ERPs), 11
intraoperative staging, 11–12
laparoscopy, 12
margins, 12–13
oncoplastic, 13
operative approach, 12
physiological tremor filtration, 12
preoperative therapy, 10–11
principles, 10
prophylactic antibiotics, use of, 11
reconstruction, 13–14
robotic, 12–13
staging, 10
techonological developments, 12
'systemic anticancer therapy' (SACT), 20

tamoxifen, 40–42, 41
tamsulosin, 37
targeted therapies, 5, 46, 48
taste changes, 67
taxanes, 29
temozolamide, 24
temporary stoma, 14
temsirolimus, 45
terazocin, 37
thermoplastic masks, 31
thoracostomy, 19
thrombocytopenia (TCP), 26, 27
thyroid cancer, 81
T-lymphocytes associated antigen 4 (CTLA4), 46
tomosynthesis, 6
topoisomerase II inhibitors, 29
total mesorectal excision (TME), 14
toxicities from TKIs and mABs, 49
toxicities of chemotherapy, 23, 32
acute, 26
cardiac, 26, 28–29
chronic, 26
GI, 27
haematological, 27
hair loss, 26
impairment of fertility, 29
late effects, 28
nausea and vomiting, 28
neurological, 28
pulmonary, 28
second cancers, 29
toxicities of radiotherapy
abdomen, 37
acute, 34
acute oesophageal effects, 36
bladder, 37
bone marrow suppression, 35
brain, 35
breast, 37
chest, 36

depletion of normal stem cells, 34
dry mouth (xerostomia), 36
fatigue, 35
gastrointestinal (GI), 37
on head and neck, 35–36
hearing impairment, 35
late, 34
moist desquamation, 35
oesophageal ulceration, 36
ovarian failure, 38
pneumonitis, 36
radiation sensitivity, 34
rectum, 37–38
skin reactions, 34
steroid, 35
of supraclavicular area, 37
swallowing dysfunction, 36
syndrome of brachial plexopathy, 37
timing of side effects, 34
urine infection, 37
vaginal stenosis and vaginal dryness, 38
toxicity of endocrine therapy, 43
transanal endoscopic microsurgery (TEM), 12
transverse abdominis muscle flap (TRAM), 13
trastuzumab, 25, 46
trastuzumab emtansine (TDM-1), 46
treatment adherence, 4
treatment intent, 2–3, 20, 21
treatment selection, factors influencing, 3
tretinoin, 46
tyrosine kinase inhibitors (TKIs), 44

ultrasound, 6

vaccines, 47
vancomycin-resistant enterococci (VRE), 5
vemurafenib, 44–45
V600E mutation, 44
vertebroplasty, 18
vinblastine, 24
vincristine, 24
vinorelbine, 24
vitamin D, 41
vomiting, 26, 28, 59, 67
radiotherapy, 37
vorinostat, 46

whole-brain radiotherapy (WBRT), 18, 35
'window of opportunity' studies, 21
work-related satisfaction, 2
World Health Organization (WHO), 79

90Y-ibritumomab tiuxetan, 46
yttrium-90 (90Y), 46

zinc supplementation, 36